Contents

Ministry of Agriculture, Fisheries and Food

Manual of Nutrition

London: Her Majesty's Stationery Office

© Crown copyright 1985
First published 1945
Ninth edition 1985

ISBN 0 11 242739 1

12 Nutritional value of meals and diets

Tables

Foreword

The ninth edition of the *Manual of Nutrition* is published at a time when there is increasing interest in the relationships between food and health. There has been particular interest in fat, sugar, salt and dietary fibre, but the science of nutrition is much broader than that. This Manual therefore describes all the important nutrients, their roles in the body, the foods that provide them, and the ways in which we digest these foods so that we can take advantage of their nutritional value.

As in the previous edition, this book then goes on to describe the effects of cooking and processing on each nutrient, and the nutritional principles involved in choosing and evaluating sensible eating habits. There are also sections on the special nutritional needs of different sections of the population and how they can be met, and finally there are appendices which give up-to-date values for the typical nutrient content of a wide range of common foods, describe UK legislation affecting the nutrient content of foods and their labelling, and give suggestions for further reading.

We are indebted to David Buss, Hazel Tyler, Sigrid Barber and Helen Crawley of the Ministry's Nutrition Branch for all their work in the preparation of this edition.

Ministry of Agriculture, Fisheries and Food
July 1985

PART 1

Nutrients and their utilization

1 Introduction to nutrition, and some definitions

The foods eaten in other countries are very different from our own, yet the majority of people grow well and stay healthy provided that they get enough to eat. The reasons for this, and the ways in which the adequacy of any diet can be assessed, form part of the science of nutrition with which this Manual is concerned. A knowledge of its principles is thus important to all of us, but especially to those who plan and provide meals.

Before proceeding further, it is necessary to define some terms:

The science **Nutrition** is the study of all processes of growth, maintenance and repair of the living body which depend upon the digestion of food, and the study of that food.

Food is any solid or liquid which when swallowed can supply any of the · following:

(a) material from which the body can produce movement, heat, or other forms of energy,

(b) material for growth, repair, or reproduction,

(c) substances necessary to regulate the production of energy or the processes of growth and repair.

Foods are considered in more detail in Part 2.

The components of foods which have these functions are called **nutrients**. They are introduced below, and considered in more detail in Chapters 2, 3, 4, 7 and 8.

The **diet** consists of those foods or mixtures of foods in the amounts which are actually eaten (usually each day). A good diet will provide adequate amounts of all the nutrients, without harmful excesses, from a wide range of foods.

The nutrients in food

The following types of nutrients may be present in foods:

Carbohydrates, which provide the body with energy, and may also be converted into body fat.

Fats, which provide energy in a more concentrated form than carbohydrates, and may also form body fat.

Proteins, which provide materials (amino acids) for growth and repair. They can also be converted into carbohydrate and used to provide energy.

Minerals, which are used in growth and repair, and help to regulate body processes.

1

Vitamins, which help to regulate body processes.[1]

Although water, like oxygen from the air, is also essential for life, it is not usually considered as a food or a nutrient. On the other hand, alcohol would be considered a food because it provides energy, even though it has drug-like properties. Iron from a cooking pot is also a nutrient since it may be used to renew substances in the blood.

Hardly any foods contain only one nutrient. Most are very complex mixtures, which consist mainly of a variety of carbohydrates, fats and proteins, together with water. Minerals and vitamins are present in very much smaller amounts. One hundred grams (g) of potatoes, for example, contain about 18 g carbohydrates, 2 g proteins, 80 g water and some dietary fibre, but less than 50 milligrams of the minerals and vitamins (and if fried they will also contain fat).

Energy

Energy is the ability to do work, and therefore means more than just vigorous activity. It can be derived from carbohydrates, fat, protein and alcohol not only in the body but also by burning them. Experiments show that almost exactly the same amount of energy is produced from, say, wheat when it is used for fuel in a railway engine (as it has been in times of glut) as when it is eaten by man. The essential difference between the two chemical processes is that in the body the energy is released gradually by a series of steps, each carefully controlled by an enzyme.[2] This energy is used to perform muscular work and to maintain body temperature and such processes as breathing, but a considerable amount is also lost as heat.

---

[1] *Vitamins* differ from hormones (which also help to regulate body processes) in that, with the exception of vitamin D, they cannot be made in the body and must therefore be supplied in the diet; hormones are always made within the body itself.

[2] *Enzymes* are special proteins, each of which accelerates the rate of a specific chemical reaction without itself being affected. They enable complex changes to occur in the body that would otherwise require more extreme conditions; without them life could not exist. Many require the presence of vitamins or minerals as 'co-factors' in order to act.

Other constituents of food

Water

Water comprises about two-thirds of the body's weight, and is the medium or solvent in which almost every body process takes place both inside and outside the cells. The need of the body for water is second only to its need for air: adults can survive for many weeks without food but for only a few days without water. Water comes from solid foods as well as from drinks (page 106), and it is lost by evaporation in the breath and sweat as well as in the urine. The balance of water retained in the body is normally very carefully regulated by the kidneys, but excessive losses can result from vomiting or diarrhoea in illness or from heavy sweating due to strenuous activity or a hot climate. Then, if water intake is not increased, dehydration may result. In temperate climates at least 1 litre (2 pints) of water or other fluid should be drunk each day; more will be needed if heavy work is done.

Dietary fibre

Some foods, particularly cereals and some fruit and vegetables, contain substantial amounts of 'dietary fibre' (roughage). In contrast to the nutrients described, this mixture of indigestible materials is not absorbed into the body; instead, it adds bulk to the faeces. This property may be beneficial to health, although fibre can also decrease the absorption of certain nutrients – especially some of the minerals. Dietary fibre is further discussed on page 7.

Flavours, colours, etc.

In addition to the main nutritive and structural components, foods also contain innumerable minor constituents which give them their characteristic flavours, colours and textures. Control over the changes which occur in these constituents after ripening, and during storage, preparation and cooking is an important part of the art of both cooks and food technologists.

Malnutrition

The maintenance of health in an individual depends upon the consumption and absorption of appropriate amounts of energy and all the nutrients. Too little or too much of some over a period of months or longer may lead to ill health or malnutrition. Although the body has considerable power to adapt to reduced dietary intakes, for example by reduced physical activity, too low an intake of food will eventually result in *undernutrition*, and, in extreme cases, *starvation*. An example is the wasting (marasmus) in young children, and stunting of physical and perhaps even mental development, which may result from inadequate breast-feeding or from a poor weaning diet in developing countries. Other examples include the 'classical' nutritional

3

deficiency diseases such as scurvy and some anaemias which result from diets containing too little of one or more minerals or vitamins, or from a physiological inability to absorb these nutrients. Equally, excessive fatness (obesity) from too great a food intake is also a form of malnutrition, as is the excessive consumption of any nutrient, whether fat, sugar, mineral or vitamin, if it leads to ill health.

Standard measurements of amount

Standard units must be used to calculate the energy and nutrients in various amounts of food, and to measure heights and weights. The metric system (including the form known as SI[1]) has mainly been used in this edition of the Manual. The relationships between these and traditional units are given in some detail in Appendix 1.

---

[1] This system mainly affects the definition of energy, which has been measured in kilo*calories* (1 kcal being the amount of heat required to raise the temperature of 1 kilogram of water by 1°C). The SI unit, the *joule*, is hard to define in familar terms, but 1 kilojoule (kJ) may be visualized as the amount of heat required to raise the temperature of 239 grams of water by 1°C. 1 Megajoule (1 MJ) = 1000kJ.

4

2 Carbohydrates

There are three major groups of carbohydrates in food: *sugars, starches,* and *cellulose and related materials.* All are compounds of carbon, hydrogen and oxygen only, and their chemical structures are all based on a common unit (nearly always glucose). The units can be linked together in different ways and in different numbers, and classification of the carbohydrates depends primarily on the number of units; this varies from one to many thousands. Sugars and starches are a major source of man's food energy throughout the world, and cellulose is one of the main constituents of *dietary fibre.*

Sugars

MONOSACCHARIDES (or simple sugars)

Glucose (dextrose) occurs naturally in fruit and plant juices and in the blood of living animals. Most carbohydrates in food are ultimately converted to glucose during digestion. Glucose can also be manufactured from starch by the action of acid or specific enzymes. *Glucose syrups* (liquid glucose) result from the partial hydrolysis of starch (usually maize or corn starch), and are mixtures of glucose, maltose and several more complex carbohydrates. Although glucose is the sugar present in the highest concentration, these syrups are always less sweet than pure glucose. They are used in many manufactured foods including sugar confectionery, soft drinks and jams.

Fructose occurs naturally in some fruit and vegetables and especially in honey. It is the sweetest sugar known. It is also a component of sucrose, from which it may be derived, and is present in commercial 'high fructose' syrups.

Galactose does not occur in the free state, but forms part of lactose.

DISACCHARIDES

Disaccharides consist of two monosaccharides linked together (minus the elements of water):

Sucrose occurs naturally in sugar cane and sugar beet, and in lesser amounts in fruits and some roots such as carrots. It is a chemical combination of glucose and fructose. 'Sugar', whether white or brown, is essentially pure sucrose.

Maltose is formed during the breakdown of starch by digestion and, for example, when grain is germinated for the production of malt liquors such as beer. It is a combination of 2 glucose units.

Lactose occurs only in milk, including human milk. It is less sweet than sucrose or glucose, and is a combination of glucose and galactose.

Table 1. **Average carbohydrate content of selected foods, g per 100 g edible portion (Available carbohydrate, as monosaccharides)**

	Sugars	Starch	Total
Milk	4.6[1]	0	4.6
Ice cream	19.7	1.0	20.7
Meat	0	0	0
Sugar	105.3[2]	0	105.3[2]
Honey	76.4	0	76.4
Jam	69.2	0	69.2
Baked beans	5.8	9.3	15.1
Potatoes, boiled	1.0	17.0	18.0
Yams, boiled	0.2	29.6	29.8
Bananas	16.2	3.0	19.2
Oranges	8.5	0	8.5
Peaches, canned in syrup	22.9	0	22.9
canned in juice	12.9	0	12.9
Biscuits, chocolate	43.4	24.0	67.4
Bread, white	2.8	45.8	48.6
Bread, wholemeal	1.8	39.8	41.6
Flour, white	0.5	76.2	76.7
Cornflakes	7.4	77.7	85.1
Muesli, average	26.2	40.0	66.2
Porridge oats	1.1	64.9	66.0
Orange squash undiluted	26.1	0	26.1
Soup, canned, tomato	2.6	3.3	5.9
Tomato ketchup	22.9	1.1	24.0
Chocolate, milk	56.5	2.9	59.4
Beer, bitter	2.3	0	2.3
Wine, medium, white	2.5	0	2.5

[1] Lactose
[2] Equivalent to 100 g of sucrose:
   1 g disaccharide is equivalent to 1.05 g monosaccharide
   1 g starch is equivalent to 1.11 g monosaccharide

The main sources of sugars in the diet are sugar, sweets and chocolates, milk (as lactose), fruit and fruit products, and biscuits and cakes. The main sources of starches in the diet are bread, potatoes, cakes, biscuits, and other cereal products.

Properties of sugars

All sugars, whether monosaccharides or disaccharides, dissolve in water and are varyingly sweet in taste. Their taste may be modified by cooking (e.g. by caramelization). They usually form white (colourless) crystals when the water in which they are dissolved becomes supersaturated, but impure preparations may be brown. In addition to providing a readily available source of energy and sweetness, sugars have other uses in foods: in jam-making, canning and freezing they act as preservatives, and in biscuits, cakes, soft drinks and some other foods they also help to provide the characteristic texture and consistency.

Non-sugar sweeteners

Some other substances also taste sweet. *Sorbitol* and *mannitol*, which are made from glucose or sucrose, are related to the sugars and are sometimes used in diabetic foods because they are absorbed only slowly; however, their energy value is similar to that of glucose. In contrast, *saccharin, aspartame* and *acesulfame K* have no chemical or nutritional relationship to sugars and provide essentially no energy. They do not rank as foods, but may be used as sweetening agents when it is desirable to restrict the amount of sugar in the diet. They are about 200-500 times as sweet as sucrose.

Starch

There are a number of starches, which are POLYSACCHARIDES composed of variably large numbers of glucose units linked together to form both straight and branched chains (*amylose* and *amylopectin* respectively). They exist in granules of a size and shape characteristic for each plant. In this form they are insoluble in water, and foods such as flour and potatoes are indigestible if eaten raw. When heated or cooked in the presence of water the starch granules swell and eventually gelatinize. They can then be more easily digested. In contrast, dry heat as in the manufacture of some breakfast cereals can make part of the starch more resistant to digestion.

Glycogen is similar to starch in composition, but is made from glucose only by animals and not by plants. Small amounts are stored in the liver and muscles as an energy reserve. It is not a significant item in the diet because it breaks down again to glucose after an animal's death.

Cellulose and related materials

These POLYSACCHARIDES provide the rigid and fibrous structure of vegetables, fruits and cereal grains (as well as wood), including the cell walls which enclose the starch granules. They are insoluble in water. Together with lignin (which is not a carbohydrate) they are the main components of *dietary fibre*.

Cellulose consists of many thousands of glucose units. It cannot be digested by man, but can be used as food by cows and other ruminants whose digestive tract contains micro-organisms capable of breaking it down into glucose. Cellulose and certain other indigestible polysaccharides add bulk to the faeces because of their water binding capacity and greatly assist the

7

passage of digestible materials and waste products through the intestines. There is much interest in the relationship between this property and human health.

Pectin is another complex polysaccharide present in apples and many other fruits and in such roots as turnips. Its property of forming a stiff jelly is important in jam-making. Pectin is not fibrous, and because it is completely digested it has little effect on the faeces, yet it is often considered as a part of dietary fibre.

Table 2. **Dietary fibre content of selected foods as measured by two different methods, g per 100 g edible portion**

	Method A	Method B
Meat	0	0
Baked beans	3.2	7.3
Beans, haricot, dry	15.1	25.4
Beans, runner	4.4	2.9
Cabbage	2.7	3.4
Carrots	2.3	2.9
Potatoes	1.3	1.8
Tomatoes	1.7	1.5
Apples	1.9	2.0
Bananas	1.1	3.4
Raisins	1.7	6.8
Nuts, hazel	4.3	6.1
Peanuts	6.0	8.1
Biscuits, digestive	2.9	5.1
Biscuits, rich tea	2.2	2.3
Bread, white	1.6	4.1
Bread, brown	4.3	6.4
Bread, wholemeal	5.8	8.5
Flour, white	2.3	4.0
Flour, wholemeal	8.9	8.1
All bran	23.7	26.0
Porridge oats	6.5	7.7
Rice Krispies	0.9	6.0
Shredded Wheat	9.8	11.2
Weetabix	9.8	9.3
Macaroni	2.6	5.5
Rice, white	0.5	3.0
Rice, brown	1.7	4.2
Spaghetti	2.7	5.6

Method A excludes 'resistant starch' while method B includes it as a part of dietary fibre. It is not yet known whether resistant starch shares all the properties attributed to dietary fibre.

The main sources of fibre in the diet are bread and flour, other cereal products, and vegetables.

Sources of carbohydrates in the diet

Plants form sugars in their leaves by the action of sunlight, but store them in their stems, roots, tubers or seeds as starch (the small amount of starch in unripe fruits, however, turns back into glucose or sucrose on ripening). Starch forms the major energy reserve of most plants, and thus in turn provides a major part of man's food energy. Sugars would hardly be present in the diet at all (except for lactose from milk and fructose from fruit and honey) were it not for the liberal use of sucrose and glucose syrups both alone and in jams, tinned fruit, cakes, biscuits, ice cream and other foods prepared in the home or by food manufacturers.

The sugar and starch content of selected foods is shown in Table 1. About one-third of the present intake of carbohydrate in the UK consists of sucrose and glucose syrups, 7 per cent is lactose, and the remainder, starch; a century ago, flour and potato consumption was much higher and sucrose consumption much lower. Then, as in the developing countries now, starch was much more important in the diet. The total fibre content of the average UK diet has not changed much over the past century, but a greater proportion now comes from fruit and vegetables and less from cereals as a result of changing eating habits. There has, however, been a recent increase in the consumption of wholemeal bread and bran-containing breakfast cereals.

Health aspects of carbohydrates

Although all sugars and starches absorbed by the body provide similar amounts of energy, they have different physiological effects. Excessive consumption of sugars and sweets is associated with increased tooth decay, especially when eaten between meals and in a form which sticks to the tooth surface, but there is more controversy about the relationship between different dietary carbohydrates and the development of obesity, heart disease, and bowel diseases such as appendicitis and bowel cancer. Nevertheless, if diets low in fat are eaten and energy intakes are to be maintained, it is wiser to increase the intake of fibre-rich starchy foods than of sugar, protein (which can be expensive) or alcohol.

Although there are no agreed recommendations for the amounts of sugars, starches or dietary fibre to be eaten by men, women or children, it is nevertheless useful to know the amounts of these constituents in different foods, so they are shown separately in Tables 1 and 2.

Some individuals, particularly of non-white races, have a limited ability to digest lactose. 'Lactose intolerance' is not usually found in infants who depend on milk, but it may develop in later life; it results in digestive disturbances when the equivalent of a glass or more of milk is drunk.

Diabetes is discussed on pages 32 and 98.

9

3 Fats

Fats include not only 'visible fats' such as butter and margarine, cooking fats and oils, and the fat on meat, but also the 'invisible fats' which occur in milk, nuts, lean meat, and other animal and vegetable foods. They are a more concentrated source of energy than carbohydrates, and are the form in which much of the energy reserve of animals and some seeds is stored.

Like carbohydrates, fats are compounds of carbon, hydrogen and oxygen only, but the proportion of oxygen is lower. Chemically, food fats consist mainly of mixtures of *triglycerides*. Each triglyceride is a combination of three *fatty acids* with a unit of glycerol (glycerine), and the differences between one fat or oil and another are largely the result of the different fatty acids in each.

Table 3. **Typical fatty acid composition of some foods as bought**

	Fat g per 100 g edible portion	Fatty acids, per cent of fat by weight[1]		
		Saturated	Monounsaturated	Polyunsaturated
Milk, cows'	3.9	64	28	3
Milk, human	4.1	48	39	8
Cheese, Cheddar	33.5	63	27	4
Eggs	10.9	31	39	11
Beef, average	27.4	41	47	4
Pork, average	25.5	35	42	15
Chicken	12.8	30	45	20
Liver, lambs	6.2	28	29	15
Mackerel	22.9	20	49	20
Butter	82.0	68	23	4
Margarine, hard	81.0	39	47	10
Margarine, soft	81.0	30	41	26
Margarine, polyunsaturated	81.0	17	27	52
Corn (maize) oil	99.9	13	25	58
Blended oil	99.9	8	52	36
Potato crisps	35.9	34	40	21
Peanuts, roasted, salted	49.0	21	38	37
Biscuits, chocolate	27.6	65	26	4
Chocolate, milk	30.3	58	33	4

[1]The total percentage of fatty acids is less than 100 because of the glycerol and other fatty compounds which are present. To calculate the total fatty acid content of a food, multiply the percentages of the various types of fatty acid by the amount of fat. Thus the total polyunsaturated fatty acid content of 100 g of beef is $\frac{4}{100} \times 27.4 = 1.1$ g.

Fatty acids

Dozens of different fatty acids are found in nature. They differ in the number of carbon atoms and 'double bonds' which they contain. *Saturated* fatty acids have no double bonds and this makes them stable, while *polyunsaturated* fatty acids have two or more double bonds which react gradually with air and make the fat rancid. All fats contain both types, as well as *monounsaturated* fatty acids, but in widely varying proportions depending on the source (Table 3). Large amounts of polyunsaturated fatty acids affect the physical as well as the chemical properties of the fats, making them liquid at room temperature (i.e., oils). Unsaturated fatty acids can be changed into saturated fatty acids and into a mixture of *cis* and *trans* monounsaturated fatty acids by controlled treatment with hydrogen (hydrogenation). This happens when liquid oils are hardened in the manufacture of margarine and in the rumen of cows and sheep. *Trans* fatty acids behave in some respects like saturated fatty acids. The more important fatty acids in foods are:

SATURATED FATTY ACIDS

Palmitic acid and *stearic acid*, which are major constituents of hard fats such as lard, suet and cocoa butter.

Butyric acid, which, although present in only small amounts in milk fat and butter, makes an important contribution to their taste. Free butyric acid is released when these fats become rancid.

UNSATURATED FATTY ACIDS

Oleic acid (monounsaturated, with one double bond) occurs in substantial amounts in all fats, and especially in olive oil where it provides 70 per cent of the total fatty acid content. *Trans* isomers of oleic acid are found in hard margarines and in lesser amounts in ruminant fats (milk, cheese, beef and lamb).

Linoleic acid (with 2 double bonds), which occurs in large amounts in vegetable seed oils such as maize (corn), soya bean and sunflower seed oils, and in small amounts in some animal fats such as pork.

Linolenic acid (with 3 double bonds), which occurs in small amounts in vegetable oils, especially linseed oil.

Arachidonic acid (with 4 double bonds), which occurs in very small amounts in some animal fats. It can be formed in the body from linoleic acid. Fatty acids with even more double bonds occur in fish oils prior to hydrogenation.

Linoleic, linolenic and arachidonic acids are called *'essential fatty acids'* because they are required in small quantities for normal health but cannot be made within the body. Once called vitamin F, enough of these fatty acids should be present in the diet to provide about 1-2 per cent of the energy intake.

Properties of fats

Fats are solid at low temperatures and become liquid when they are heated. Oils are simply fats which are liquid at room temperature, usually as a result of their higher content of unsaturated fatty acids, and will solidify on refrigeration as with olive oil. Oils and fats do not dissolve in water, but may be *emulsified* with water by vigorous mixing as when butter and margarine are made. Emulsions usually separate unless emulsifiers such as lecithin from soya beans or egg are added.

Fat makes an important contribution to the texture and palatability of many foods. Furthermore, because it is digested comparatively slowly, foods rich in fat have a high satiety value (page 28).

Food fats usually contain small amounts of other fat-soluble substances, including flavour components and some of the vitamins. Animal fats may contain retinol (vitamin A) and vitamin D, and varying amounts of cholesterol, while vegetable fats may contain carotenes (which can be converted into vitamin A in the body) and vitamin E, but no cholesterol.

The amount of energy obtained from all common fats is about the same, despite the different functions and properties of many of the component fatty acids.

Mineral oils such as liquid paraffin, are chemically different from food fats and oils despite their similarity in appearance. They cannot be utilized by the body, but function as laxatives and will reduce the absorption of some nutrients.

Sources of fat in the diet

Vegetable sources In plants, fats are formed from carbohydrate. Thus, when seeds such as sunflower and cottonseed ripen, their starch content decreases as their fat content rises. Oilseeds such as these and groundnuts (peanuts), coconuts, rapeseeds, palm kernels and soya beans contain about 20-40 per cent of oil; they are among the chief sources of fat for the manufacture of margarine. The fat content of flour and other cereal products apart from oatmeal is generally low, as is the fat content of most vegetables and fruits. The proportion of each fatty acid present varies from plant to plant, and is also quite variable within a species. It can sometimes be altered by genetic breeding.

Animal sources Animals, including man, store excess energy almost entirely in deposits of fat, the amount of which is very variable. As in plants, this fat can be made from carbohydrate – but the dietary carbohydrate can be starch, sugar or even (in cows and sheep) cellulose. Animals also lay down fat from their dietary fat; in this case the fatty acid composition reflects that of the diet, except for ruminants whose digestive processes normally make the fatty acids more saturated.

Fish such as herring, mackerel, pilchards, salmon, sardines, tuna and eels are sometimes called *fatty fish*; the proportion of fat in them varies with the season of the year. *White fish* such as cod, haddock and plaice contain little fat except in the liver. Fish liver is also a rich source of vitamins A and D. The fat content of many foods, especially meat, varies widely. Average values, and the main sources of fat in the UK diet, are shown in Table 4. The amount of fat in the diet tends to be higher in more affluent families and countries. In Britain and in most other developed countries, fat has for many years provided about 40 per cent of the energy value of the diet, but less than 10 per cent is derived from fat in many of the world's poorest countries.

The average proportion of polyunsaturated to saturated fatty acids (the 'P/S ratio') in the whole diet is about 0.3:1, having risen from about 0.2:1 in 1970.

Table 4. **Average fat content of foods as bought, g per 100 g edible portion**

Milk, whole	3.9	Fish, white, filleted	0.9
Milk, semi-skimmed	1.7	Mackerel	22.9
Milk, skimmed	0.1	Tuna, canned in oil	22.0
Yogurt, low fat, fruit	0.7	Butter	82.0
Ice cream	8.2	Margarine	81.0
Cheese, Cheddar	33.5	Low fat spread	40.7
Cheese, Edam	22.9	Vegetable oils	99.9
Cheese, cottage	4.0	Lard and dripping	99.1
Eggs	10.9	Potatoes	0.2
Beef, average	27.4	Chips, fried	10.2
Lamb, average	25.6	Chips, oven, baked	4.2
Pork, average	25.5	Peanuts, roasted	49.0
Bacon, streaky	37.3	Bread, white	1.7
Sausages, pork	32.1	Bread, wholemeal	2.5
Chicken	12.8	Porridge oats	9.2
Turkey	6.0		

The main sources of fat in the diet are fats and oils including butter and margarine, meat and meat products, and milk.

Health aspects of fats

Diets in poor countries are often low in energy, and the United Nations have recommended an increase in fat intakes to raise their nutritional value. Conversely, the United Nations and other bodies have recommended a decrease in the fat content of the diets of affluent populations as a means of reducing the risk of heart disease. In the UK, the Department of Health and Social Security has recommended that those adults and children over 5 years old for whom fat provides more than 35 per cent of their energy intake, or for whom saturated and *trans* fatty acids (page 11) together provide more than 15 per cent of their energy intake, should adjust their diet until these

13

values are reached. Although no change is recommended in the intake of polyunsaturated fatty acids, some increase may nevertheless be necessary if the diet is to remain palatable.

Examples of the necessary calculations are given on pages 100 and 118, although it must be recognised that these recommendations strictly apply only to the diet as a whole over a long period. Calculations of this type can be misleading when applied to individual foods or meals.

High concentrations of cholesterol in the blood are associated with an increased risk of coronary heart disease. High intakes of saturated fatty acids can increase this cholesterol in susceptible individuals, but cholesterol in food has little or no effect: the liver compensates for any deficiency by making its own.

4 Proteins

All proteins are compounds of carbon, hydrogen and oxygen, but, unlike carbohydrates and fats, they always contain nitrogen as well. Most proteins also contain sulphur and some contain phosphorus. They are essential constituents of all cells, where they regulate the processes of living or provide structure. Protein must be provided in the diet for the growth and repair of the body, but any excess is used to provide energy.

Proteins consist of chains of hundreds or even thousands of amino acid units. Only about 20 different amino acids are used, but the number of ways in which they can be arranged is almost infinite. It is the specific and unique sequence of these units which gives each protein its characteristic structural and enzymatic properties.

Amino acids

It is convenient to divide amino acids into two types: *essential* and *non-essential*. *Essential* amino acids cannot be made in the body, at least in amounts sufficient for health, and must therefore be present in the food. *Non-essential* amino acids are equally necessary as components of all proteins in the body; they differ only in that it is possible for them to be made from any excess of certain other amino acids in the diet.

The 8 amino acids essential for *adults* are:

Isoleucine	Phenylalanine
Leucine	Threonine
Lysine	Tryptophan
Methionine	Valine

and another amino acid, histidine, is also essential for the rapidly growing *infant*.

The remaining amino acids which are widespread in proteins are:

Alanine	Glycine
Arginine	Proline
Aspartic acid	Serine
Cysteine	Tyrosine
Glutamic acid	

Animal and vegetable proteins

The overall proportions of amino acids in any single vegetable food (cereals, nuts and seeds, potatoes, or legumes such as peas and beans) differ from those needed by man. For example, wheat is comparatively low in lysine, maize is low in tryptophan, and legumes are low in methionine (Table 5). These proteins are therefore said to have low *biological values*, because the *quality* of a protein depends on its ability to supply all the essential amino acids in the amounts needed. Mixtures of such foods, however, complement each other and result in greatly enhanced values.

Most animal proteins (from meat, fish, milk, cheese and eggs) have a high biological value. The reason for this is that man is part of the animal kingdom; the proteins of animals are therefore more like those of man and can be utilized by us with the minimum of waste. In effect, animals have pre-selected with varying degrees of efficiency the plant amino acids which they and we need and have burned up the remainder for energy (page 31). Nevertheless, the nutritional advantages of animal foods over vegetable foods in practice lie more in the presence of associated nutrients such as vitamin B_{12}, iron and vitamin D than in the protein.

Because there is no way in which excesses of amino acids can be stored in the body, they will be most efficiently used if a complete assortment is supplied to the body at about the same time. This can be achieved by eating a mixed diet at each meal – and provided that the total energy content of the diet is also adequate. Mixtures of vegetable protein foods such as beans on toast or of animal and vegetable protein foods such as fish and chips, bread and cheese, and breakfast cereals with milk, therefore have a sound physiological basis.

Texturized vegetable proteins

Because animals convert plant protein into their own muscle slowly and inefficiently (only 5-10 per cent being retained), ways have been developed to concentrate or isolate the proteins from a number of plants, especially soya

Table 5. **Proportion of some essential amino acids in selected proteins, g per 100 g protein**

	Lysine	Methionine	Tryptophan
Milk, cows'	8.0	2.8	1.4
Eggs	6.2	3.2	1.8
Beef	9.1	2.7	1.3
Beans, soya	7.0	1.4	1.4
Peanuts	4.1	1.3	1.3
Wheat[1]	2.8	1.7	1.2
Maize[1]	3.0	2.1	0.7

[1] Some amino acids can be increased by genetic breeding.

beans, and convert them *directly* into products which resemble meat. Such vegetable protein products, if suitably fortified with the most important minerals and vitamins which meat provides, such as thiamin, riboflavin, vitamin B_{12}, iron and zinc, can be used instead of meat and are acceptable to vegetarians (vegetarian diets are discussed on page 97).

It is also possible to utilize micro-organisms such as yeasts and fungi, or otherwise inedible leaves, to provide protein-rich foods for animals and man.

Protein as a source of energy

The amount and type of protein in the diet will not exactly balance the requirements for growth, repair and maintenance: there will always be excesses of some amino acids, and usually an excess of total protein. These will be converted into glucose in the liver or be directly oxidized to provide heat and energy. Furthermore, if the energy available from the diet is insufficient to meet demands, this oxidation of the amino acids tends to take preference over their more fundamental use for rebuilding proteins. This is why it is important to ensure that diets contain sufficient energy in the form of carbohydrate and fat before expensive proteins are added, for only then can these proteins be properly utilized for those purposes for which no other nutrient can be substituted.

Other health aspects of proteins

Newborn infants can absorb some proteins intact from their mothers' milk, including antibodies which provide protection from infection. Susceptible individuals can also react to certain other food proteins: for example, those with coeliac disease react to gluten and others may react to cows' milk protein.

Some beans including red kidney beans and soya beans contain proteins which are harmful unless well cooked.

Properties of proteins

Some proteins dissove in water and some in salt water, but some do not dissolve. This is exploited in the preparation of wheat gluten which is used to improve the baking quality of home-produced wheats, when other proteins as well as starch are washed from the flour. The wheat starch may be dried and used in foods for people with coeliac disease.

The action of heat on proteins is complex. Proteins such as the albumen in egg white harden or coagulate irreversibly when heated, but are still readily digested. Individual amino acids are little affected by normal cooking procedures, although some lysine may react with carbohydrates in the food (e.g., in the baking of bread) and methionine may sometimes be reduced. In the preparation of gelatin, however, when connective tissue from meat is boiled for many hours, *all* the tryptophan is destroyed.

The brown discoloration which sometimes develops during prolonged storage of concentrated or dried milk or dehydrated vegetables is due to complex reactions between lysine and the sugars of these foods (the Maillard reaction).

Sources of protein in the diet

About one-third of the protein in the average UK diet comes from plant sources and two-thirds from animal sources. The amount of protein in nuts and dried peas and beans is very high – about the same as in meat, fish and cheese. The proportion is diluted when these legumes are soaked in water, but they remain an excellent source of good quality protein. Cereals are also rich in protein; indeed wheat, maize and rice are the main sources of protein for many people in the world. The amount of protein in most root vegetables is small, but potatoes provide useful quantities; green and leafy vegetables, however, contain insignificant amounts. The concentration of protein in selected foods is shown in Table 6.

Table 6. **Average protein content of foods as bought, g per 100 g**

Milk, whole	3.2	Baked beans	4.8
Milk, skimmed	3.4	Beans, red kidney, dry	22.1
Cheese, Cheddar	26.0	Beans, soya, dry	34.1
Cheese, feta	16.5	Peas, frozen	5.7
Beef, average	16.6	Potatoes	2.0
Lamb, average	16.2	Apples	0.3
Pork, average	16.9	Peanuts, roasted	24.3
Sausages, pork	10.6	Bread, white	8.2
Chicken	19.7	Bread, wholemeal	9.0
Turkey	22.0	Flour, white	9.4
Fish, white	17.1	Cornflakes	8.6
Prawns	22.6	Spaghetti	12.0

The main sources of protein in the diet are meat, milk, bread and other cereals.

5 Energy needs and food consumption

Uses of energy

Energy, i.e., the ability to do work, is obtained from food by controlled oxidation of the carbohydrates, fat, protein and alcohol in the diet. It is necessary for three purposes: (a) to maintain life, (b) for voluntary activities, and (c) for special purposes such as growth, pregnancy and lactation. If more is obtained than is used in these ways, the excess can be stored in the body as fat tissue.

MAINTENANCE OF LIFE

Energy is required for breathing, the heartbeat, the maintenance of body temperature, and other involuntary activities including brain function. The amount needed can be measured in people at complete rest or asleep. The rate of this *basal* or *resting metabolism* is higher in relation to body size in infants and actively growing young children than in adults. After adolescence, the needs are proportional to the amount of lean tissue in the body; thus women tend to have lower resting metabolic rates than men both because they are lighter and because muscle generally forms a lower proportion of their body weight (and fat a higher proportion). The rate is also lower in old people, or in starvation, because of the reduction which occurs in lean tissue. It is thus possible to adapt to changed energy intakes.

After food is eaten, extra heat is produced and more energy is needed to cover this. The amount varies with the food. Climate does not significantly affect the resting metabolism, but the rate does vary widely between apparently similar individuals because the efficiency of the body processes varies. Some average values are:

	Weight kg	Resting energy requirement kcal(MJ)/day	kcal(MJ)/kg/day
Infant, 1 year old	10	500 (2.1)	50 (0.21)
Child, 8 years old	25	1,000 (4.2)	40 (0.17)
Adult woman	55	1,300 (5.4)	25 (0.1)
Adult man	65	1,600 (6.7)	25 (0.1)

19

A man therefore needs about 1 kilocalorie (nearly 5 kilojoules) each minute just to keep alive. During 8 hours sleep, the resting requirement of 400-500 kcal (1.7-2.1 megajoules) is all that would be used, but during the remainder of the day the additional requirements of physical activity must be taken into account.

ACTIVITY

Whenever people move, they use extra energy. The heavier they are the more it takes, and strenuous activities of course require more energy than light ones. There are also substantial variations between apparently similar individuals. It is easier to measure the total energy expended (*including* the resting metabolic energy) during any activity than it is to measure the supplement for that activity, and some examples of these totals are shown for an *average 25 year old man* weighing 65 kg (10 stone):

	Average energy expenditure	
Everyday activities	kcal/min	kJ/min
Sitting	1.4	6
Standing	1.7	7
Washing, dressing	3.5	15
Walking slowly	3	13
Walking moderately quickly	5	21
Walking up and down stairs	9	38

Work and recreation

Light
Most domestic work		
Golf		
Lorry driving	2.5-4.9	10-20
Light industrial and assembly work		
Carpentry, bricklaying		

Moderate
Gardening		
Tennis, dancing, jogging		
Cycling up to 20 km per hr	5.0-7.4	21-30
Digging, shovelling		
Agricultural work, non-mechanized		

Strenuous
Coal mining, steel furnace work	7.5 and	
Squash, cross-country running	over	Over 30
Football, swimming (crawl)		

Additional energy is needed during *growth* to provide for the extra body tissue. However, even in rapidly growing children the amount is small in comparison with the needs for maintenance and movement.

During pregnancy and lactation, all the infant's needs for energy (as for other nutrients, see page 93) must be supplied by the mother. Up to 80,000 kcal (335 MJ) of extra food energy may be needed during a *pregnancy*, mostly during the final months. Some of this is used to build up a store of about 4 kg of fat in the mother which may be gradually drawn upon during *lactation*, but an additional intake of 600 kcal (2.5 MJ) per day from the diet is also recommended at this time (page 56).

Total energy requirements

The dietary energy required by an individual who is neither gaining nor losing weight exactly equals the energy expended on maintenance and physical activity. In practice this balance is achieved over periods of a few days, with remarkable accuracy: an excessive intake of only 10 kcal each day would be equivalent to a weight gain of about 1 lb (0.5 kg) every year.

The energy expended during a day can be estimated from the average values given above, taking into account the times spent on different leisure and occupational activities. Thus, a male sedentary worker such as a civil servant might expend 2,510 kcal (10.5 MJ) in a typical day, as follows:

	kcal	MJ
8 hr asleep at 1.1 kcal per min	530	2.2
8 hr at work		
6 hr sitting at 1.4 kcal per min	500	2.2
2 hr standing and walking averaging 2.5 kcal per min	300	1.2
8 hr non-occupational activities		
2 hr 15 min travelling, averaging 1.7 kcal per min	230	0.9
15 min washing and dressing, at 3.5 kcal per min	50	0.2
1½ hr light domestic activities, averaging 3 kcal per min	270	1.2
3 hr sitting, eating, reading, watching television, at		
1.4 kcal per min	250	1.1
30 min squash, averaging 7.5 kcal per min	230	0.9
30 min gardening, averaging 5 kcal per min	150	0.6
Total energy expenditure	2,510	10.5

Because of individual variations, the diet of any particular sedentary worker may provide more or less energy than this; the average intake of a group of such people would, however, be expected to be close to this value.

In summary, the daily energy requirement of any adult is that amount which maintains the desirable body weight. Energy requirements depend on:

Body size and composition Heavy people use more energy for maintenance and physical activity, although some may spend less time than lighter people in activities. Women tend to need less energy than men, although their needs are increased during pregnancy and lactation.

Age Requirements for maintenance are *proportionately* highest in infants and young children, and lowest in old people who have less lean body tissue and are less active.

Physical activity The degree of activity is the most important factor in determining energy requirements, and also the most difficult to assess. Sedentary workers (clerical and professional people, drivers and many shop assistants) need a total of about 900 kcal (3.8 MJ) for 8 hours work; moderately active people (many industrial workers, railwaymen, postmen and bus conductors) need about 1,200 kcal (5.0 MJ) and very active workers (miners at the coal face, and some building labourers, farm workers, dockers, and army recruits) have an average need for about 1,800 kcal (7.5 MJ) during 8 hours at work. Leisure activities such as jogging, particularly if indulged regularly or for long periods, also affect the day's requirements.

Obesity

If an individual eats or drinks foods which provide more energy than he uses up in his daily activity, some of the fat, protein, carbohydrate or alcohol will be converted into body fat. Any kind of food can therefore be 'fattening'. Some foods, however, are more concentrated sources of energy than others, or their palatability is such that excessive amounts are more likely to be eaten; these tend to be foods containing little water and a high proportion of fat or sucrose, such as butter, margarine and fried foods, and sugar, sweets, cakes and biscuits. Alcoholic drinks in excess can also lead to obesity, as appetite, which normally limits food intake, appears to restrict drinking somewhat less.

Life insurance companies have calculated acceptable weights for people of different heights, their interest arising from the toll taken by obesity-related diseases including coronary heart disease, diabetes and complications arising during surgery. The values in Table 7 are *not* increased during middle and old age.

Obesity may be defined as a weight more than 20 per cent above the upper end of the ranges shown.

Weight may be lost by decreasing energy intake or increasing physical activity, or both. Conversely, weight may be gained by increasing energy intake or decreasing physical activity. The exact consequences of these changes are difficult to predict because of the large differences between individual responses and some measure of adaptation, but for most people the part played by changes in activity is likely to be comparatively small. For example, if a man trying to lose weight takes a brisk half hour walk, he will expend about 100 kcal (420 kJ) more than if he sat watching television. If at the end of his walk he is thirsty and drinks a pint of beer, he will take in substantially more energy than he used up and should not be surprised if his weight increases. Nevertheless, *regular* exercise can be an important factor in weight control.

Table 7. Acceptable weight ranges for men and women

	Height (without shoes)			Weight (without clothes)	
	ft	in	cm	lb	kg
Men	5	5	165	121-152	55-69
	5	6	168	124-156	56-71
	5	7	170	128-161	58-73
	5	8	173	132-166	60-75
	5	9	175	136-170	62-77
	5	10	178	140-174	64-79
	5	11	180	144-179	65-80
	6	0	183	148-184	67-83
	6	1	185	152-189	69-86
	6	2	188	156-194	71-88
	6	3	191	160-199	73-90
Women	4	11	150	94-122	43-55
	5	0	152	96-125	44-57
	5	1	155	99-128	45-58
	5	2	157	102-131	46-59
	5	3	160	105-134	48-61
	5	4	163	108-138	49-62
	5	5	165	111-142	51-65
	5	6	168	114-146	52-66
	5	7	170	118-150	53-67
	5	8	173	122-154	55-69
	5	9	175	126-158	58-72
	5	10	178	130-163	59-74

Prepared from data published in the Royal College of Physicians' Report on Obesity, 1983.

Anorexia

It is important to realise that some body fat is essential for health, but a few people, particularly teenaged girls, seek to reduce their weight below the desirable range in Table 7. *Anorexia nervosa* is the name given to extreme measures including starvation and vomiting sometimes used to achieve this, and it can be fatal.

Energy value of food

The energy provided by the fat, protein and carbohydrate in food, and by alcohol, can be measured. Taking into account the small proportions of these nutrients which are not absorbed into the body, it is accepted that:

1 g dietary carbohydrate (calculated as monosaccharides) provides 3.75 kcal or 16 kJ

1 g dietary fat provides 9 kcal or 37 kJ

1 g dietary protein provides 4 kcal or 17 kJ

1 g alcohol provides 7 kcal or 29 kJ

Small amounts of energy can also be derived from organic acids such as citric acid in fruits and drinks and acetic acid in vinegar. Minerals, vitamins and, of course, water do not provide energy.

The energy value of any food can be calculated when the proportion of these nutrients in it are known. For example each 100 g of potato crisps contain 6.3 g protein, 35.9 g fat and 49.3 g carbohydrate, so the energy content is calculated as follows:

$$
\begin{aligned}
6.3 \times\ 4 &=\ \ 25.2 \text{ kcal from protein} \\
35.9 \times\ 9 &= 323.1 \text{ kcal from fat} \\
49.3 \times\ 3.75 &= 184.9 \text{ kcal from carbohydrate} \\
\hline
\text{Total} &\quad 533.2 \text{ kcal}
\end{aligned}
$$

or

$$
\begin{aligned}
6.3 \times 17 &=\ \ \ 107.1 \text{ kJ from protein} \\
35.9 \times 37 &= 1{,}328.3 \text{ kJ from fat} \\
49.3 \times 16 &=\ \ \ 788.8 \text{ kJ from carbohydrate} \\
\hline
\text{Total} &\quad 2{,}224.2 \text{ kJ}
\end{aligned}
$$

It is misleading, however, to imply that energy values can be obtained with such precision; decimal points should not be included in the results, which might be rounded to 533 kcal or 2,224 kJ. But when performing further calculations such as for the proportion of energy derived from fat, it is wiser to use the detailed figures and round off only at the end:

$\dfrac{323.1}{533.2} \times 100 = 60.60$ or 61 per cent of energy from fat.

Sources of energy in the diet

Nearly all the weight of any food is made up of protein, fat and carbohydrate together with water. Foods which contain large amounts of water, such as salad vegetables, fruit and clear soups will contain little protein, fat or carbohydrate, and consequently provide little energy. In contrast, dry foods such as breakfast cereals, and foods rich in fat (each gram of which provides more than twice as much energy as each gram of protein or carbohydrate) will be excellent sources of energy. The main sources of energy in the UK diet are bread, flour and other cereals, meat, visible fats, dairy produce and sugar

– foods which are not only rich in energy but also eaten in substantial quantities. For some people, sweets and alcoholic drinks are also a significant source of energy. The energy (and water) contents of selected foods are shown in Table 8.

Table 8. **Average energy value and water content of selected foods, g per 100 g edible portion**

	Energy		Water
	kcal	kJ	g
Milk, whole	65	272	88
semi-skimmed	45	191	89
skimmed	32	137	91
Cheese, Cheddar	406	1,682	37
Yogurt, low fat, fruit	89	382	77
Beef, average	313	1,296	55
Bacon, streaky	387	1,599	46
Chicken	194	809	67
Fish, white	77	324	82
Sardines, canned in oil, drained	217	906	58
Eggs	147	612	75
Butter/margarine	735	3,020	16
Low fat spread	366	1,506	51
Vegetable oil	899	3,696	0
Sugar	394	1,680	0
Courgettes	29	122	92
Lettuce	12	51	96
Mushrooms	13	53	92
Potatoes	74	315	79
Chips	234	983	44
Apples	46	196	84
Bananas	76	326	71
Dates, dried	248	1,056	15
Oranges	35	150	86
Bread, white	230	977	38
Flour, white	337	1,437	14
Biscuits, chocolate	524	2,197	2
Cornflakes	368	1,567	3
Crispbread, rye	321	1,367	6
Beer, bitter	37	156	93
Wine, white, medium	89	371	85
Spirits	222	919	68

The significance of hot foods

The heat of hot food is trifling compared with the energy provided by metabolism of its constituents within the body. For example, the constituents of tomato soup provide 55 kcal per 100 g; a serving of 250 ml (9 oz) would therefore provide about 140 kcal. The additional heat provided by its cooling from a serving temperature of, say, 60°C to the body temperature of 37°C would be about 6 kcal. Nevertheless, this heat is immediately perceived, and gives a useful boost to morale on cold days.

6 Digestion of food and absorption of major nutrients

Food has been defined as any solid or liquid which, when swallowed, can provide the body with energy, or material for growth and repair, or certain substances for regulating body processes. However, it is clear that almost any food can be recovered virtually intact from the stomach if vomiting occurs soon after it is eaten. Therefore, food cannot really be said to have entered the body until it has been:

(a) *Digested*, i.e., physically and chemically broken down into simple component parts which can be

(b) *Absorbed*, i.e., passed through the walls of the digestive tract into the blood (or lymph).

Flavour and appetite

For food to be eaten, it must be appetizing or we must be hungry or preferably both circumstances apply. When and how much we eat is determined by a number of factors.

The complex sensation of *hunger* occurs when the body's energy stores are reduced (giving rise to reduced levels of glucose and fatty acids in the blood) and the stomach is empty. But people, especially obese people, do not eat only when they are hungry and stop when they cease to feel hungry. *Appetite* is a sensation which relates to the smell and taste of particular foods and their ingredients, and is influenced by the surroundings, habits, and emotional state of the individual, all of which can also increase or decrease the flow of saliva and other digestive juices. Thus, where there is freedom of choice, more attractive food is more likely to be eaten, and it can be seen that good cooking and pleasant surroundings are important in nutrition. It should, however, be noted that some appetizing foods such as confectionery products can be relatively low in many nutrients, and that unappetizing foods can provide nourishment if they are eaten – as when an unconscious person is fed through a stomach tube.

The process of digestion

Although cooking softens meat fibres and the cellulose of plant materials, and gelatinizes starch, true digestion only begins when food enters the digestive tract. The digestive tract is illustrated in the diagram; it is basically a tube about 5 metres long.

Diagram of digestive system

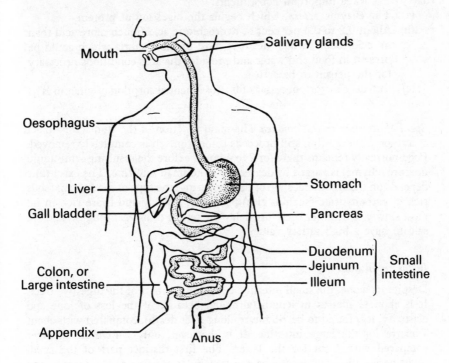

In the mouth

(a) Food is mechanically broken down by chewing. It is therefore important to have healthy teeth and gums.

(b) The food is mixed and moistened with saliva.

Saliva comes from salivary glands under the tongue and at the back of the mouth. It is usually present in the mouth, but its flow is increased by the smell and taste of food and by chewing. It helps the food to be swallowed, and also contains an enzyme, ptyalin, which converts a small amount of the starch into maltose.

In the stomach

After the mixture of food particles and saliva has been swallowed – the final voluntary action – it takes about 3 seconds to pass down the oesophagus (gullet) into the stomach, where:

(a) The food is mixed with gastric juice.

(b) More mechanical breakdown results from stomach contractions.

Gastric juice is produced by the lining of the stomach in response to the same

27

stimuli that increase saliva flow. Normally, about 3 litres are produced each day. It has three important constituents:

(a) The enzyme *pepsin*, which begins the digestion of protein.
(b) About 0.2 to 0.4 per cent of hydrochloric acid (much more acid than in 'acid foods') which destroys most of the bacteria which could be present in food and water and provides the acid conditions necessary for the pepsin to be active.
(c) 'Intrinsic factor', necessary for subsequent absorption of vitamin B_{12}.

Speed of digestion in the stomach The main function of the stomach is to act as a reservoir: digestion still proceeds if the stomach is completely removed. Food normally remains there for 2 to 4 hours before the resulting semi-liquid mixture (chyme) is passed by degrees into the small intestine. The exact time depends on the emotional state of the person and the type of food eaten: foods rich in carbohydrate (such as rice) pass most quickly and those rich in fat most slowly. The latter therefore delay the return of hunger longest, and are said to have a high satiety value.

In the small intestine

Despite its name, the small intestine is the longest part of the digestive tract. It is about 3 metres in length (although because of the loss of tone and elasticity, it is found to be 7-8 metres long after death), compared with about 1 metre for the large intestine. It is, however, only 2-4 cm in diameter compared with 6 cm for the latter. The first distinct part of the small intestine is called the *duodenum*; the remainder consists of the *jejunum* and finally the *ileum*. It is in this organ that the main part of both digestion and absorption takes place.

In the duodenum, the digestive juices poured on to the food mixture from three sources are:

(a) *Bile*, which is produced in the liver and stored in the gall bladder. Bile salts emulsify the fat into microscopic droplets so that it can be digested.
(b) *Pancreatic juice*, from the pancreas. This alkaline liquid neutralizes the acid chyme, and contains a number of enzymes for breaking down fats, proteins and carbohydrates into their component parts. The most important of these are *lipase* which splits fatty acids from the triglycerides of fat, *trypsin* and *chymotrypsin* which split proteins into small peptides and amino acids, and *amylase* which splits starch into maltose.
(c) *Intestinal juice*, from the walls of the small intestine itself. This also contains digestive enzymes.

The final phase of digestion occurs *in* the intestinal wall after absorption, when peptides are split into their component amino acids, maltose is converted into glucose by *maltase*, sucrose into glucose and fructose by *sucrase*, and lactose into glucose and galactose by *lactase*.

In the large intestine

Substances which have resisted digestion thus far can be used for food by the bacteria present in the large intestine (colon). Some cellulose and other components of dietary fibre may then be broken down, and the bacteria will form B-vitamins and vitamin K which provide small amounts of additional nutrients for absorption. They also generate gas (mainly hydrogen).

Table 9. **Summary of the major enzymes of digestion**

	Where active	Action
Pytalin (from saliva)	Mouth	Some starch to maltose
Pepsin	Stomach	Protein to peptides
Rennin (in infants only)	Stomach	Milk protein to peptides
Trypsin (from pancreas)	Intestine	Protein to peptides and amino acids
Chymotrypsin (from pancreas)	Intestine	Protein to peptides and amino acids
Lipase (from pancreas and intestine)	Intestine	Fat to fatty acids
Amylase (from pancreas)	Intestine	Starch (and glycogen) to maltose
Maltase	Intestinal wall	Maltose to glucose
Sucrase	Intestinal wall	Sucrose to glucose and fructose
Lactase	Intestinal wall	Lactose to glucose and galactose

Digestion in infants

Before birth, infants are nourished through their bloodstream via the mother's placenta. The change to intestinal digestion does not develop fully for several months. Three consequences in particular may be noted:

(a) For a few days, some whole proteins can be absorbed without digestion. In this way, antibodies against some diseases may be absorbed intact from the mother's milk.

(b) The stomach contains the enzyme *rennin*, which clots the casein of milk and begins its digestion.

(c) Starch cannot readily be digested until the infant is several months old.

Indigestion

A food or food component is indigestible if it cannot be fully broken down into substances capable of absorption. Some, such as lactose from milk in lactose-intolerant individuals, will reach the large intestine and be fermented by the bacteria present; this results in the production of gas and diarrhoea. Indigestion also means discomfort or pain in the gastro-intestinal tract resulting from eating. It can result as much from emotional factors as from the passage of indigestible foods.

The process of absorption

In the mouth

No significant absorption occurs through the lining of the mouth.

In the stomach

The following simple substances can pass through the lining of the stomach into the blood stream in *small* quantities:
  (a) Water
  (b) Alcohol
  (c) Sugars
  (d) Minerals which are soluble in water, such as salt
  (e) Vitamins which are soluble in water, i.e., B-vitamins (but not vitamin B_{12}, which can only be absorbed in the ileum with the aid of the intrinsic factor produced by the stomach) and vitamin C.

In the small intestine

Almost all the absorption of nutrients occurs through the walls of the small intestine. Most of the water, alcohol, sugars, minerals, and water-soluble vitamins are absorbed here too, as well as the digestion products of the energy producing nutrients – that is:
  (a) Peptides and amino acids from proteins
  (b) Fatty acids from fats
  (c) Disaccharides from starch
Fat-soluble vitamins are absorbed in association with the fatty acids.

Absorption into the cells of the intestinal wall is remarkably efficient; indeed, more than half of the small intestine can be removed without major consequences. The surface of the wall contains innumerable projections, called *villi*, which present a very large surface area (20-40 square metres in total) for absorption. This process occurs both passively (by diffusion) and actively (when specific nutrients are drawn into cells already containing large amounts of those nutrients).

Absorption can, however, be impaired. In coeliac disease the villi are lost, and substances such as laxatives and dietary fibre which speed the passage of the intestinal contents may reduce absorption in general. The fibre and phytic acid present in wholemeal cereals may also reduce the absorption of specific minerals including calcium, iron and zinc.

In the large intestine

The main functions of the large intestine are to absorb water from the residue moving through it from the small intestine, and to store the resultant faeces until they are expelled through the anus. Faeces contain the indigestible materials of food, but consist mainly of debris from the continuously replaced cells of the intestinal wall. The entire passage of food from mouth to anus takes from 1 to 3 days, but it can be decreased by disease or by antibiotics which kill the intestinal bacteria, or it can be increased to as long as a week by diets very low in dietary fibre.

The fate of major nutrients in the body

Carbohydrates

The disaccharides entering the intestinal wall are split into monosaccharides which are carried by the bloodstream directly to the liver. They may then be:

(a) Passed as glucose to all the cells of the body to be used directly for energy via a series of controlled steps which also produce carbon dixoide and water.

(b) Converted into glycogen and stored in the liver and skeletal muscles as a readily available source of energy.

(c) Converted into fatty acids and stored in the body fat (adipose tissue) as a source of energy.

The hormone *insulin* is required before glucose can enter cells, but fructose (and dietary sorbitol, which is converted in the body into fructose) does not require insulin for its metabolism.

Fats

Almost all the fatty acids which enter the intestinal wall are immediately rebuilt into triglycerides which are carried to the bloodstream by lymph. Fat, in the form of microscopic particles called *chylomicrons*, gives the blood plasma a milky appearance for some time after a large meal is eaten. Fat may be further transformed by the liver, and is finally deposited in the adipose tissue. This reservoir of fat is constantly available as a source of energy via another series of controlled steps which also give rise to carbon dioxide and water.

Proteins

When the peptides enter the intestinal wall they are split into amino acids which are carried in the blood directly to the liver. Then:

(a) They may be passed into the general circulation where they enter the body's 'pool' of essential and non-essential amino acids. These are then built into the structural proteins and specific enzymes which each cell needs.

(b) The excess of some amino acids may be converted into certain others.

(c) The residual excess of amino acids is oxidized for energy, in some cases after conversion into glucose. Urea is also formed and excreted through the kidneys. If the diet as a whole is inadequate in energy, then a greater proportion of the protein will be used for this purpose in order to keep the body alive.

Control of nutrients in the blood

Blood is the means by which most nutrients are carried to and from the cells where they are needed. The concentration of most nutrients in the blood is normally controlled automatically as described in chapter 7 and 8. In addition, when carbohydrate is eaten, the resulting slight increase in blood glucose is soon reduced by the hormone insulin. In *diabetes*, however, the pancreas does not secret sufficient insulin, and the blood glucose concentration increases until the excess is excreted by the kidneys into the urine. In 'insulin-dependent' diabetes, the symptoms resulting from this imbalance are so severe that insulin must be injected, but other forms of diabetes can usually be controlled by dietary regulation leading to a reduction in body weight.

7 Minerals

Most if not all of the inorganic elements or minerals can be detected in the body, but only about 15 of them are known to be essential and must be derived from food. Minute amounts of a further 5 or more are necessary for normal life in other animal species, and may well prove to be necessary for man; it is difficult, however, to conceive of a dietary deficiency of these.

Minerals have three main fuctions:
   (a) As constituents of the bones and teeth. These include *calcium, phosphorus* and *magnesium.*
   (b) As soluble salts which help to control the composition of body fluids and cells. These include *sodium* and *chlorine* in the fluids outside the cells (e.g., blood), and *potassium, magnesium* and *phosphorus* inside the cells.
   (c) As essential adjuncts to many enzymes, and other proteins such as haemoglobin which are necessary for the release and utilization of energy. *Iron* and *phosphorus*, and most of the other elements described at the end of this chapter, act in this way.

The seven elements above are the best understood, and are in general needed in the greatest amounts in the diet or are present in the largest amounts in the body tissues (Table 10); these, together with sulphur which is mainly present as part of the amino acids methionine and cysteine, may be considered as the *major minerals*. The remainder, including cobalt, copper, chromium, fluorine, iodine, manganese, selenium and zinc, are equally essential but needed in smaller or much smaller quantities; they are called *trace elements*. A large excess of most of these can be poisonous.

MAJOR MINERALS

Iron

Function, and effects of deficiency

Healthy adults contain about 3 to 4 g of iron, more than half of which is in the form of haemoglobin, the red pigment of blood. Iron is also present

Table 10. **Daily intake and total body content of minerals for a reference man**

	Daily intake		Total body content	
Major minerals				
Calcium	1.1	g	1,000	g
Phosphorus	1.4	g	780	g
Sulphur	0.85	g	140	g
Potassium	3.3	g	140	g
Sodium	4.4	g	100	g
Chlorine	5.2	g	95	g
Magnesium	0.34	g	19	g
Iron	16.0	mg	4.2	g
Trace elements				
Fluorine	1.8	mg	2.6	g
Zinc	13.0	mg	2.3	g
Copper	3.5	mg	72	mg
Selenium	0.15	mg	>15	mg
Iodine	0.2	mg	13	mg
Manganese	3.7	mg	12	mg
Chromium	0.15	mg	Less than 2 mg	
Cobalt	0.3	mg	1.5 mg	

Intakes are generally likely to be far greater than requirements. A variable proportion is actually absorbed into the body (ranging from almost 100 per cent for sodium and chlorine down to about 5-10 per cent for iron, copper, manganese and probably chromium and cobalt too); the amount absorbed normally balances the amount lost in urine and sweat, except where increased retention is necessary during growth.

in the muscle protein myoglobin, and is stored to some extent in organs such as the liver. This store is an important source of iron for the first 6 months of an infant's life because the amount of iron in milk is small. Iron is involved with the use of oxygen: haemoglobin transports oxygen from the lungs to the tissues, and other iron-containing substances utilize the oxygen within the cells.

If food provides insufficient iron to replace the body's losses, the stores are gradually depleted. Eventually anaemia results. Anaemia can also arise from a number of other causes including deficiencies of folic acid and vitamin B_{12}; cures are best effected medically and not nutritionally, for example by the use of iron salts which can be absorbed in much larger amounts than the iron from food.

Absorption and excretion

The amount of iron in the body is controlled almost entirely by the amount absorbed, because losses occur only when blood or other whole cells are lost in the general wear and tear of life. Losses do not occur at the end of the red blood corpuscles' life of 3-4 months, because the iron from them is efficiently re-utilized.

The absorption of iron from food is generally low, but is increased when the body's stores are depleted and when needs are greatest as in growing children or menstruating or pregnant women. Iron is most readily absorbed from meat including offal (up to 25 per cent). Less than 5 per cent of the other forms of iron such as those in eggs and vegetables or added to flour is absorbed; the exact amounts depend on other factors in the diet, e.g., it is increased by vitamin C but decreased by the tannins in tea.

Sources

About a fifth of the iron in the British diet comes from meat. The total amounts of iron present in selected foods is shown in Table 11.

Table 11. **Total iron content of selected foods, mg per 100 g edible portion**

Milk, whole	0.1	Aubergine	0.4
Eggs	2.0	Cabbage	0.6
Beef, average	1.9	Potatoes	0.4
Corned beef	2.4	Watercress	1.6
Chicken	0.7	Yam	0.3
Kidney, pigs	6.4	Apricots, dried	4.1
Liver, lambs	7.5	Bread, white	1.6
Fish, white	0.5	Bread, wholemeal	2.7
Curry powder	29.6	Cornflakes, fortified	6.7
Soy sauce	4.8	Cocoa powder	10.5
		Chocolate, plain	2.4
		Wine, red	0.8

The main sources of iron in the diet are meat, bread, flour and other cereal products, potatoes and vegetables.

Calcium

Function, and effects of deficiency

Calcium is the most abundant mineral in the body. All but about 1 per cent of it is in the bones and teeth, together with more than three-quarters of the body's phosphorus, as calcium phosphates deposited in an organic framework. In addition to giving strength to the bones, these minerals act as a reserve supply for other needs and the calcium is constantly withdrawn into and replaced from the blood at carefully controlled rates. The remaining 5-10 g of calcium are essential for the contraction of muscles including the heart muscle, for nerve function, for the activity of several enzymes, and for normal clotting of the blood.

Too little calcium *in the bodies* of young children results in stunted growth and in rickets (where the leg bones are deformed); in women who lose large quantities of calcium through repeated pregnancies and lactation and in some old people the deficiency may show as osteomalacia (decalcified bones). Old people, especially women, also frequently develop osteoporosis (loss of bone). However, in Britain these diseases are unlikely to be caused by low levels of calcium *in the diet* for the body can normally adapt to these; the primary deficiency in rickets and osteomalacia is of vitamin D, so that too little calcium is absorbed (page 51), while the basic cause of osteoporosis is still unknown.

Absorption and excretion

Only 20-30 per cent of the calcium in the diet is normally absorbed and the remainder is lost in the faeces. But without adequate amounts of vitamin D, little or no calcium can be absorbed, and when dietary fibre or phytic acid (present mainly in the outer layers of cereals) is added to the diet, calcium absorption is also reduced. It was partly to compensate for this that calcium carbonate was added to the high extraction flour used during and after World War II; it is still added to all flour except wholemeal even though it is now known that the body can adapt to the presence of phytic acid.

Excretion of the absorbed calcium is mainly through the kidneys, and is increased when the diet contains large amounts of protein; some calcium is also lost in sweat. Adults normally absorb enough calcium to balance these losses until middle age unless they are immobilized, but pregnant and lactating women and growing children who are forming new bone must of course obtain more.

Sources

Few foods besides milk and cheese and, in Britain, most bread (page 80) contain significant amounts of calcium, as shown in Table 12. It is therefore important that these foods are included in the diet, especially for children and pregnant and lactating women whose needs are greatest.

Table 12. **Calcium content of selected foods, mg per 100 g edible portion**

Milk, whole	103	Aubergine	10
Milk, evaporated	260	Cabbage	57
Milk, dried skimmed	1,230	Onions	31
Yogurt, low fat, natural	200	Potatoes	8
Cheese, Cheddar	800	Watercress	220
Eggs	52	Apples	4
Beef, average	7	Figs, dried	280
Fish, white	22	Peanuts, roasted	61
Sardines, canned in oil	550	Bread, white	105
(fish only)		Bread, wholemeal	54
		Rice	4

The main sources of calcium in the diet are milk, cheese, bread and flour (if fortified) and green vegetables. For some people, hard water and the bones in canned sardines and salmon can be important sources.

Phosphorus

Phosphorus is the second most abundant mineral in the body and, in the form of various phosphates, has a wide variety of essential functions. Calcium phosphates provide the strength of the bones and teeth, and inorganic phosphates are a major constituent of all cells. Phosphates play an essential role in the liberation and utilization of energy from food. They are also constituents of nucleic acids and some fats, proteins and carbohydrates, and must be combined with some B-vitamins in the body before the latter can be active.

Because phosphorus is present in nearly all foods, dietary deficiency is unknown in man. Furthermore, phosphates are added to a number of processed foods. It should, however, be noted that high intakes of phosphorus in the first few days of life may produce low levels of calcium in the blood, and muscular spasms (tetany). This can result from the use of unmodified cows' milk which has a high ratio of phosphorus to calcium compared with human milk, and in which the calcium may combine with the fat present and be poorly absorbed.

Table 13. **Phosphorus and magnesium content of selected foods, mg per 100 g edible portion**

	Phosphorus	Magnesium
Milk, whole	88	10
Cheese, Cheddar	520	25
Eggs	220	12
Beef, stewing steak	140	18
Chicken	170	21
Ham	313	19
Fish, white	171	23
Cabbage	54	17
Potatoes	38	17
Oranges	24	13
Peanuts, roasted	370	180
Bread, white	79	20
Bread, wholemeal	210	76
Chapati, made without fat	120	37
Marmite	1,700	180

The main sources of phosphorus in the diet are milk and milk products, bread and other cereal products, and meat and meat products. The main sources of magnesium are milk, bread and other cereal products, potatoes, and other vegetables.

Magnesium

Most of the magnesium in the body is present in the bones, but it is also an essential constituent of all cells and is necessary for the functioning of some of the enzymes which are involved in energy utilization.

Magnesium is widespread in foods, especially those of vegetable origin because it is an essential constituent of chlorophyll. Less than half is normally absorbed and, unlike the chemically related element calcium, this

37

process is unaffected by vitamin D. Deficiency is rare, and results from excessive losses in diarrhoea rather than from low intakes.

Sodium and chlorine

Functions, and effects of deficiency and excess

All body fluids contain salt (sodium chloride), but especially those outside the cells such as blood. These elements are involved in maintaining the water balance of the body, and sodium is also essential for muscle and nerve activity.

Salt requirements are closely related to water requirements, and too low an intake results in muscular cramps. Salt intake may, however, have to be severely restricted in certain kidney diseases or where there is marked water retention. Very young infants also cannot tolerate high sodium intakes because their kidneys cannot excrete the excess, so salt should not be added to infants' diets. Habitually high salt intakes are associated with high blood pressure.

Absorption and excretion

It is essential for life that the concentration of sodium and chloride in the blood is maintained within close limits. As an excess of (added) salt in the diet is readily absorbed, control of sodium in the blood is achieved by its excretion through the kidneys into the urine. There is also a variable loss through sweat. This is only significant after strenuous exercise or in hot climates, as for miners in deep pits, steel workers and athletes; although adaptation can occur, extra salt may still be needed to prevent muscle cramps.

In a temperate climate the amount of salt needed by an adult is less than 3 g per day, although this amount could be lost in the sweat in 2 hours of strenuous activity in the sun. Such an intake can be achieved from the salt already present in food, but most people add much more and take in from 5 to 20 g per day.

Sources

Sodium and chlorine are comparatively low in all foods which have not been processed, but salt is added to very many prepared foods. For example salt, is low in pork and other fresh meats but high in bacon, sausages, and most other meat products; low in herrings but high in kippers. Salt is also added to canned vegetables and most butter, margarine, cheese, bread and some breakfast cereals during manufacture, and to many foods during home cooking and on the plate. Sodium may also be derived from sodium bicarbonate and monosodium glutamate.

Potassium

Function, and effects of deficiency

Potassium is present largely in the fluids within the body cells where its concentration is carefully controlled. The total amount in the body can be measured, and is closely related to the amount of lean tissue. Potassium has a complementary action with sodium in the functioning of cells.

As with sodium, most of the potassium in the diet is absorbed and the excess is excreted through the kidneys. Losses may be large if diuretics or purgatives are frequently taken, and in protein-energy malnutrition (kwashiorkor) where tissue breakdown as well as diarrhoea occurs. In severe cases of potassium depletion, heart failure may result unless supplements are given.

Table 14. **Sodium and potassium content of some foods as bought, mg/100 g edible portion**

	Sodium	Potassium
Milk, whole	50	140
Cheese, Cheddar	610	120
Eggs	140	136
Beef, average	70	330
Corned beef	854	134
Pork, average	65	360
Bacon, streaky	1,245	183
Chicken	75	290
Sausages, pork	760	160
Haddock, fresh	120	300
Haddock, smoked	1,220	290
Butter, salted	780	15
Butter, unsalted	12	15
Margarine	800	5
Potatoes	8	360
Potato crisps	550	1,190
Cauliflower	8	350
Peas, frozen	3	190
Peas, canned, processed	380	150
Tomatoes	3	290
Orange juice/oranges	2	180
Canned peaches	1	150
Raisins	52	860
Bread, white	525	110
Bread, wholemeal	560	230
Cornflakes	1,160	99
Weetabix	360	420
Coffee, instant	81	3,780
Marmite	4,500	2,600
Chocolate, milk	120	420
Soy sauce	5,720	270

The sodium content of vegetables is much higher if they are cooked in salted water. Apart from this, the main sources of sodium in the UK diet are table salt, bread and cereal products, meat products including bacon and ham, and milk. The main sources of potassium are vegetables, meat and milk. Fruit and fruit juices are also noteworthy as being much richer in potassium than sodium.

TRACE ELEMENTS

Knowledge of the exact roles and dietary requirements for some of the following minerals is incomplete for three reasons: they have only recently been found to be essential; dietary deficiencies of many are unknown; and the utilization of one may be affected by the amounts of other elements present.

Cobalt

Cobalt can be utilized by man only in the form of vitamin B_{12} (page 48).

Copper

Copper is associated with a number of enzymes. Deficiency has occasionally been observed in malnourished infants, particularly if their initial stores were depleted by prolonged feeding of cows' milk alone (which contains less copper than most foods). Although shellfish and liver are particularly rich in copper, the main sources in the average diet are meat, bread and other cereal products, and vegetables. Excessive copper can be poisonous.

Chromium

Chromium is involved in the utilization of glucose. It is fairly widely distributed in foods.

Fluorine

Fluorine is associated with the structure of bones and teeth, and increases the resistance of the latter to decay. Drinking water is an important source, but the natural content is variable and is often below the optimum level of 1 mg per litre (1 part per million). The only other important sources of fluorine in the diet are tea, sea-food (especially fish whose bones are eaten) and, if eaten, fluoridated toothpaste!

Iodine

Iodine is an essential constituent of hormones produced by the thyroid gland in the neck, and most of the iodine in the body is in this gland. Deficiency causes it to enlarge – a condition known as goitre. The most reliable source of iodine is sea-food. The amount of iodine in vegetable and cereal foods depends on the level in the soil, and that in animal foods depends on the level in their diet. Because of the widespread use of iodides in animal feed milk is now the main source of iodine in the British diet, and milk products, meat and eggs are also important. The use of iodized table salt is beneficial in areas where goitre is prevalent, whether it results from low intakes of iodine itself or from reduced absorption caused by goitrogens in vegetables from the cabbage family.

40

Manganese

Manganese is associated with a number of enzymes. Tea is exceptionally rich in manganese, and plant products, including nuts, spices and whole cereals are in general much better sources of manganese than are animal products.

Selenium

Selenium is needed for an enzyme in the red blood cells, and the main dietary sources are meat, fish and cereal products. The selenium content of plants varies widely with the level in the soil, and in some parts of the world animals fed on local produce develop symptoms of deficiency or excess. Neither is common in man, especially in Britain where our food comes from a wide variety of sources.

Zinc

Zinc helps with the healing of wounds, and is also associated with the activity of a wide variety of enzymes; nevertheless most of the comparatively large amount which is present in the body is in the bones. Zinc is present in a wide variety of foods, particularly in association with protein, and meat and dairy products are thus excellent sources. Less than half of the zinc in the diet as a whole is absorbed, and absorption is further reduced if large amounts of whole cereals rich in dietary fibre and phytic acid are eaten; this is as likely a cause of deficiency (resulting in stunting) as is a low intake *per se*, and may put some vegetarians at risk.

Table 15. **Zinc content of selected foods, mg per 100 g edible portion**

Milk	0.4
Cheese, Cheddar	4.0
Beef, stewing steak	3.8
Chicken	1.1
Fish, white	0.4
Eggs	1.5
Potatoes, old	0.3
Bread, white	0.6
Bread, wholemeal	1.8
Chapati, made without fat	1.0

The main sources of zinc in the diet are meat and meat products, milk, bread, and other cereal products.

8 Vitamins

Until the beginning of the 20th Century, it was believed that the only components of a diet necessary for health, growth and reproduction were pure proteins, fats, carbohydrates and a number of inorganic elements. This view had to be changed when it was found that minute amounts of additional materials were also essential. These factors could be extracted from a variety of foods and appeared to be of two types: fat-soluble ('A') and water-soluble ('B'). They were later each discovered to contain several active components, or vitamins. The former mainly associated with fatty foods, is now known to include vitamins A, D, E and K. The vitamin B complex includes thiamin (B_1), riboflavin (B_2), niacin (or nicotinic acid), folic acid, vitamin B_6, vitamin B_{12}, biotin and pantothenic acid. Vitamin C is also water-soluble, but occurs in different foods from the B-vitamins. Many of these vitamins exist in more than one chemical form.

The absence of a vitamin from the diet, or, more commonly in practice, its presence in insufficient amounts, leads to both general and specific symptoms. The most common general symptoms are, as with deficiencies of many other things, a feeling of malaise and restriction of the growth of children. The specific symptoms of deficiency in man are discussed separately for each vitamin. Excessive intakes of most water-soluble vitamins, either from vitamin pills or from very unusual diets, have very little effect as they are rapidly excreted in the urine, but excessive intakes of fat-soluble vitamins accumulate in the body and can be dangerous.

Factors affecting the stability of the vitamins in foods are discussed elsewhere (page 67).

Vitamin A

The chemical name of vitamin A is *retinol*. Retinol itself is found only in animal foods, but milk and some vegetable foods also contain the deep yellow or orange *carotenes* which can be converted in the body to retinol and are therefore sources of vitamin A activity. The most important of these is beta(β)-carotene. The most convenient way of expressing the total vitamin A activity of a diet is as *retinol equivalents:* by definition, 1 μg retinol equivalent is equal to 1 μg retinol or 6 μg β-carotene[1]. This average value takes into account the conversion losses and the lesser absorption of β-carotene compared with retinol in the general diet.

Function, and effects of deficiency or excess

Vitamin A is essential for vision in dim light; thus prolonged deficiency (sufficient to deplete any stores in the liver, which in previously well nourished people will last for 1 to 2 years) results in night blindness. In children in many parts of the world deficiency also results in severe eye lesions (xerophthalmia) and complete blindness (keratomalacia). Vitamin A is also necessary for the maintenance of healthy skin and surface tissues, especially those which excrete mucus.

Excessive doses, for example from taking large amounts of vitamin A preparations for long periods, accumulate in the liver and can be poisonous.

Sources

Vitamin A is not widely distributed in food. Fish liver oils are by far the most concentrated natural source of retinol, but animal liver, kidney, dairy produce and eggs also contain substantial amounts; lard and dripping, however, contain none. Variable amounts of β-carotene are found in carrots and dark green or yellow vegetables, roughly in proportion to the depth of their colour; thus dark plants such as spinach contain more than cabbage, and the dark outer leaves of a cabbage contain more than the pale inner heart. Furthermore, all margarine for retail sale is required by law to contain about the same amount of vitamin A as butter. This is now added in the form of synthetic retinol and β-carotene.

The amounts of vitamin A in selected foods are shown in Table 16. The British diet as a whole provides on average about twice the recommended intake of vitamin A, with two-thirds coming from retinol itself and the remaining third from carotene.

---

[1] The amounts of vitamin A in foods are sometimes quoted in international units (i.u.). To convert these to μg retinol equivalents, multiply the i.u. of retinol (in animal foods) by 0.3, and divide the i.u. of β-carotene (in plant foods) by 10. (This is because 1 i.u. vitamin A = 0.3 μg retinol or 0.6 μg β-carotene; and 1 μg retinol equivalent = 1 μg retinol or 6 μg β-carotene.)

Table 16. **Vitamin A content of selected foods, $\mu g/100$ g edible portion**

Animal foods	Retinol	
Milk	56[1]	
Cheese, Cheddar	363[1]	
Eggs	190	
Beef	10	
Liver, lambs	19,900[1]	
Kidney, pigs	160	
Cod	2	
Mackerel	45	
Sardines, canned, fish only	7	
Butter	985[1]	
Margarine	800[1]	
Cod liver oil	18,000	
Halibut liver oil	900,000	

Vegetable foods	β-carotene[2]	Retinol equivalents
Potatoes	0	0
Cabbage	300	50
Spinach	6,000	1,000
Peas, fresh or frozen	300	50
Watercress	3,000	500
Carrots, old	12,000	2,000
Tomatoes	600	100
Sweet potato	4,000	670
Apricots, dried	3,600	600
Mango	1,200	200
Flour	0	0

[1] Retinol equivalent, including carotene.
[2] β-carotene content of many vegetables and fruit varies widely depending on variety and season.

The main sources of vitamin A in the diet are liver, carrots, milk, margarine and butter.

B-Vitamins

Although the chemical structure of each of the B-vitamins is quite different, they have several features in common. They act as 'co-factors' in different enzyme systems in the body; they tend to occur in the same foods; and, being water-soluble, they are not stored for long in the body. These characteristics mean that diets containing too little of the B-vitamins can lead to *multiple* deficiency diseases within a few months.

Thiamin (Vitamin B$_1$)

Function, and effects of deficiency

Thiamin is necessary for the steady and continuous release of energy from carbohydrate. Thiamin requirements are thus related to the amount of carbohydrate, and more or less to the amount of energy, in the diet. The deficiency disease, beriberi, results from a diet which is not only poor in thiamin but also rich in carbohydrate (or alcohol), such as one based almost entirely on polished rice from which the thiamin-rich seedcoat has been removed.

Sources

Thiamin is widely distributed in both animal and vegetable foods. Rich sources are those which contain more than 0.04 mg per 100 kcal (0.01 mg per 100 kJ), such as milk, offal, pork, eggs, vegetables and fruit, whole grain cereals and fortified breakfast cereals. It should, however, be noted that cooking may result in considerable losses from these foods (page 67). Fats, sugars and alcoholic drinks contain no thiamin at all.

Wheat in the form of bread has long been a major source of carbohydrate in the British diet, but much of the thiamin is removed with the bran in the milling necessary to produce the popular white bread. Thus a 1 oz slice of wholemeal bread provides 0.10 mg thiamin (0.13 mg per 100 kcal), while 1 oz of unfortified white bread would provide about 0.03 mg thiamin (0.04 mg per 100 kcal). It is therefore a legal requirement in the UK that all flour except wholemeal be *fortified* with thiamin to at least 0.24 mg per 100 g, equivalent to 0.07 mg per 100 kcal (page 80).

Table 17. **Thiamin content of selected foods**

	mg/100 g edible portion	mg/100 kcal
Milk	0.05	0.06
Bacon, streaky	0.45	0.13
Beef, stewing steak	0.06	0.03
Corned beef	0	0
Chicken	0.11	0.06
Pork chop	0.57	0.17
Sausages, pork	0.04	0.01
Sugar	0	0
Peas, frozen	0.32	0.48
Pototoes	0.20	0.27
Soya beans, dry	1.10	0.27
Oranges	0.10	0.29
Pineapple, fresh	0.08	0.17
Peanuts, roasted	0.23	0.04
Bread, white	0.21	0.09
Bread, wholemeal	0.34	0.13
Chapati, made without fat	0.23	0.11
Cornflakes, fortified	1.80	0.49
Rice	0.41	0.11
Marmite	3.10	1.80
Beer, bitter	0	0

The main sources of thiamin in the diet are bread and cereal products, potatoes, milk, and meat.

Riboflavin (Vitamin B₂)

Function, and effects of deficiency

Riboflavin is a bright yellow substance, which is essential for the utilization of energy from food. Specific deficiency signs are rarely seen in man, but include sores in the corners of the mouth.

Sources

Although riboflavin is widely distributed in foods, especially animal foods, about one-third of the average intake in Britain is derived from one source alone – milk. As riboflavin will be destroyed by ultra-violet light, it is very important that bottled milk is not allowed to stay too long on the doorstep.

Table 18. **Riboflavin content of selected foods, mg per 100 g edible portion**

Milk	0.17
Cheese, Cheddar	0.50
Beef, stewing steak	0.23
Chicken	0.13
Liver, lambs	4.64
Kidney, pigs	2.58
Eggs	0.47
Potatoes	0.02
Sweet potatoes	0.06
Yam	0.03
Bread, white	0.06
Breakfast cereal, fortified	1.60
Wheatgerm	0.61
Tea, dry	0.90
Marmite	11.0

The main sources of riboflavin in the diet are milk, meat, fortified cereal products, and egg.

Niacin

Function, and effects of deficiency or excess

Nicotinic acid and nicotinamide are two forms of another B-vitamin (known collectively as niacin) which is involved in the utilization of food energy. Deficiency results in pellagra, in which the skin becomes dark and scaly especially where it is exposed to light. Pharmacological doses of nicotinic acid (but not nicotinamide) can cause burning sensations in the face and hands.

Sources

Two anomalies occur with pellagra: it occurs when the diet consists largely of maize, a cereal which contains nicotinic acid, and it can be cured by milk or eggs which are not rich sources of this vitamin. The reasons are firstly, that the nicotinic acid in maize and other cereals is largely present in a bound form which is unavailable to man (although it can be released by alkali as in the preparation of Mexican tortillas), and secondly, that proteins of milk and eggs are especially rich in tryptophan – an amino acid which can be converted to nicotinic acid in the body.

It is therefore convenient to express the niacin content of foods in terms of equivalents: on average *1 mg of niacin equivalent equals 1 mg of available niacin or 60 mg of tryptophan,* and this is accepted as a definition. The amounts of both forms in selected foods are shown in Table 19.

Table 19. **Niacin equivalents in selected foods, mg per 100 g edible portion**

	Niacin (total)	Tryptophan	Niacin equivalent[1]
Milk	0.1	47	0.9
Cheese, Cheddar	0.1	367	6.2
Beef, stewing steak	4.2	258	8.5
Pork chop	4.2	180	7.2
Chicken	5.9	221	9.6
Fish, white	2.9	189	6.0
Eggs	0.1	217	3.7
Beans, mung, dry	2.0	210	5.5
Peas, frozen	1.6	58	2.6
Potatoes	0.6	52	1.5
Bread, white	1.6	102	2.3[2]
Bread, wholemeal	4.1	108	1.8[2]
Wheatgerm	5.8	318	5.3[2]
Tea, dry	6.0	0	6.0
Coffee, instant	24.8	186	27.9

[1] Available niacin + (tryptophan ÷ 60).
[2] Naturally occurring nicotinic acid is considered unavailable.
The main sources of niacin in the diet are meat and meat products, potatoes, bread, and fortified breakfast cereals.

Vitamin B₆ (Pyridoxine)

Function, and effects of deficiency

Vitamin B_6, or pyridoxine, is involved in the metabolism of amino acids, including the conversion of tryptophan to nicotinic acid; the requirements are thus related to the protein content of the diet. The vitamin is also necessary for the formation of haemoglobin. Deficiency is rare in man, but women who are pregnant or taking oral contraceptives may benefit from increased intakes of this vitamin. Very high intakes, however, are dangerous.

Sources

Vitamin B_6 occurs widely in food, especially in meats and fish, eggs, whole cereals and some vegetables.

Table 20. **Vitamin B_6 content of selected foods, mg per 100 g edible portion**

Milk	0.06
Beef, stewing steak	0.27
Chicken	0.29
Turkey	0.44
Fish, white	0.29
Baked beans	0.12
Brussels sprouts	0.28
Peas, frozen	0.10
Potatoes	0.25
Oranges	0.06
Bananas	0.51
Bread, white	0.07
Bread, wholemeal	0.12
Wheat germ	0.95

The main sources of vitamin B_6 in the diet are potatoes and other vegetables, milk and meat.

Vitamin B_{12}

Function, and effects of deficiency

Vitamin B_{12} is a mixture of several related compounds, all of which contain the trace element cobalt. With folic acid, it is needed by rapidly dividing cells such as those in the bone marrow which form blood. Deficiency leads to a characterstic (pernicious) anaemia and the degeneration of nerve cells. Because vitamin B_{12} does not occur in vegetable foods, deficiency may occur in vegans who consume no meat, milk, eggs, or any special supplement, but it more usually arises in those few individuals whose gastric juice contains no 'intrinsic factor' (page 28) and who therefore cannot absorb this vitamin.

Sources

Vitamin B_{12} occurs only in animal products and in micro-organisms including yeast. Liver is the richest source, but useful amounts also occur in eggs, cheese, milk, meat and fish, and in fortified breakfast cereals, as shown in Table 21.

Table 21. **Vitamin B_{12} content of selected foods, μg per 100 g edible portion**

Milk	0.4
Cheese, Cheddar	1.5
Eggs	1.7
Beef, lamb, pork	2.0
Liver, lambs	54.0
Liver, pigs	23.0
Fish, white	2.0
Cornflakes, fortified	1.7
Marmite	0.5

The main sources of vitamin B_{12} in the diet are offals, other meat and meat products, and milk.

Folic acid

Function, and effects of deficiency

Folic acid, or folate, has several functions, including its action with vitamin B_{12} in rapidly dividing cells. Deficiency leads to a characteristic (megaloblastic) form of anaemia which must be distinguished from that caused by a deficiency of vitamin B_{12}. Folic acid deficiency can arise not only from a poor diet, as with some elderly people, but also because of increased needs for the synthesis of red blood cells in pregnant women and premature infants, and when there is decreased absorption of folic acid in gastro-intestinal disease or when some anti-epileptic drugs are given.

Sources

Folic acid occurs in small amounts in many foods, but is especially rich in offal and raw green leafy vegetables. Most fruits, meat and dairy produce contain little. Folic acid is readily destroyed in cooking, much being lost in the water used for cooking vegetables, and it is also readily oxidized to unavailable forms of the vitamin. Thus care should be taken to include good sources of folic acid in the diet to minimize the risk of deficiency.

Pantothenic acid

Pantothenic acid is necessary for the release of energy from fat and carbohydrate. Dietary deficiencies of this vitamin are unlikely in man because it is so widespread in food. Animal products, cereals and legumes are especially rich sources.

Biotin

Biotin is also essential for the metabolism of fat. Very small amounts are required, and sufficient may well be made by the bacteria normally inhabiting the large intestine. It is therefore probable that no additional biotin need be provided in the diet, except in the very unusual situation when large quantities of raw eggs are consumed: raw, but not cooked, egg white contains a substance (avidin) which combines with biotin making it unavailable to the body.

Rich sources of biotin include offal and egg yolk. Smaller amounts are obtained from milk and dairy products, cereals, fish, fruit and vegetables.

Vitamin C (Ascorbic acid)

Function, and effects of deficiency

Vitamin C is necessary for the maintenance of healthy connective tissue. Man is one of the few animals (along with monkeys and the guinea pig) unable to form his own vitamin C, and must therefore obtain it from food.

Deficiency soon results in bleeding, especially from small blood vessels and into the gums, and wounds heal more slowly. Scurvy follows, and, if the deficiency is prolonged, death results. Mild deficiencies may occur in infants who are given unsupplemented cows' milk, in people eating poor diets (particularly the elderly), and in food faddists eating little but whole cereals which contain no vitamin C.

Claims that extremely large amounts of vitamin C (10-100 times the recommended intake) prevent or cure colds and other minor ailments have little scientific basis.

Sources

Vitamin C is not widely distributed in foods. Small amounts occur in milk, especially breast milk, and liver, but virtually all the vitamin C in most diets is derived from vegetables and fruit. As many of these are comparatively expensive when out of season, and since vitamin C is readily lost from them during storage, preparation and cooking (page 67), this vitamin remains one of the few nutrients in which British diets can be deficient.

The average vitamin C content of selected foods is shown in Table 22.

Table 22. **Vitamin C content of selected foods, mg per 100 g edible weight**

	Vitamin C	Vitamin C after boiling mg per 100 g
Aubergine	5	3
Brussels sprouts	90	40
Cabbage	55	20
Cauliflower	60	20
Lettuce	15	
Pepper, green	100	
Plantain (green banana)	14	
Potatoes – new	16	9
Oct-Dec	19	9
Jan-Feb	9	6
Mar-May	8	5
Sweet potatoes	25	14
Tomatoes	20	
Apples	5	
Bananas	10	
Blackcurrants	200	150
Grapefruit	40	
Lemon juice	50	
Mango	80	
Oranges	50	

The main sources of vitamin C in the diet are potatoes, fruit juice, citrus fruit, and green vegetables. The vitamin C content of many vegetables and fruit varies widely, depending on variety, season and freshness.

Some less commonly eaten fruits such as rose hips are even richer than blackcurrants or citrus fruits, but for practical reasons their extracts are usually fortified with the equally valuable synthetic vitamin C. Vitamin C may also be added to other fruit juices to compensate for the losses which occur during storage.

The amount of vitamin C in any particular fruit or vegetable may differ considerably from the value shown in the table. This is because of the natural variations which occur, the variable losses during the time between harvesting and consumption in the home, and the variations in cooking methods that may be used. As an example, fresh peas may contain between 10 and 30 mg per 100g; the higher values would tend to occur in the spring and early summer when the plants are growing most rapidly, and may be preserved by freezing. The loss which can occur after harvesting is illustrated in Table 22 by the average change in composition of potatoes through the year; it can also be substantial in the days which elapse between the harvest of leafy vegetables and their consumption in the home. Vitamin C, like riboflavin, is also rapidly lost when milk is allowed to stand on the doorstep; this may be important for young children and those old people with restricted diets for whom milk may be one of the few sources of this vitamin.

The highest single contribution to vitamin C intake in the UK is made by potatoes (page 77), for the large amounts eaten more than compensate for the comparatively low content of this vitamin. The only vegetable materials containing no vitamin C are cereal grains (unless they are allowed to sprout) and dried peas and beans; instant potato also contains very little unless it has been fortified.

Vitamin D

Function, and effects of deficiency and excess

Vitamin D is necessary for maintaining the level of calcium (and phosphorus) in the blood. It achieves this primarily by enhancing the absorption of dietary calcium from the intestine, and by helping to regulate the interchange of calcium between the blood and bone.

Infants and children who obtain too little vitamin D develop rickets, with deformed bones which are too weak to support their weight. Because these changes readily become permanent, it is important to prevent their development; hence in the UK and some other countries vitamin D preparations are provided for children and pregnant women, and margarine and many milk products are fortified. Some adolescents and women who are repeatedly pregnant and who breast-feed all their babies, and some old people, may also suffer from bone softening (osteomalacia) because they absorb too little calcium from a diet which is low in both calcium and vitamin D.

Too high an intake of vitamin D causes more calcium to be absorbed than can be excreted; the excess is then deposited in, and damages, the kidneys. It is therefore necessary for vitamin D intakes to be carefully controlled, especially in young children.

Sources

Vitamin D is obtained both from the action of sunlight on a substance in the skin, and from the diet. Sunlight is by far the most important source for most people, who will need little or no extra from food. But two groups of people should ensure that their food contains sufficient vitamin D: firstly, children and pregnant and lactating women, whose requirements are especially high, and secondly, people who are little exposed to sunlight such as the housebound elderly and people in northern latitudes or those who prefer to wear enveloping clothes.

Few foods contain vitamin D. All those which do so naturally are animal products, and contain vitamin D_3 (cholecalciferol) derived as in humans from the action of sunlight on the animal's skin or from its own food. There may thus be seasonal variations in the amounts present. Vitamin D_3 is also used to fortify a number of foods, as (sometimes) is vitamin D_2 (ergocalciferol), which appears to be equally effective in man and can readily be manufactured from plant materials. Vitamin D is required by law in margarine for retail sale (page 72), and is also included in the supplements provided (free to those in need) in the UK for pregnant and lactating women and for children up to 5 years old.

Table 23. **Vitamin D content of selected foods, μg per 100 g edible portion**

Milk, whole	0.03
Milk, skimmed	0
Milk, skimmed, fortified	0.08
Evaporated milk	4.0
Cheese, Cheddar	0.3
Yogurt, fortified	2.0
Eggs	1.6
Beef, average	0
Liver, average	0.8
Herring and kipper	22.4
Salmon, canned	12.5
Sardines, canned	7.5
Butter	0.8
Margarine	7.9
Vegetable oil	0
Cornflakes, fortified	2.8
Ovaltine, dry	8.7
Cod liver oil	212.5

The main sources of vitamin D in the diet are, on average, margarine, fatty fish, eggs, breakfast cereals, and butter.

Vitamin E

Function, and effects of deficiency

A number of related *tocopherols* show vitamin E activity, the most active being alpha(α)-tocopherol. In rats it is necessary for normal fertility, but neither this nor many other wondrous properties ascribed to it have been proved in man. Because vitamin E occurs widely in foods, especially in those eaten by the poorest of the world's peoples, and because (like other fat-soluble vitamins) it is stored in the body, deficiency is only likely in premature infants who have very low fat stores; when fed on formulas low in vitamin E and rich in the readily oxidized polyunsaturated fatty acids (which appear to increase the need for this vitamin), an anaemia may develop. Excessive intakes do not appear to be toxic.

Sources

Most foods contain vitamin E. The richest sources are vegetable oils, cereal products and eggs; animal fats and meat, fruit and vegetables contain comparatively little.

Vitamin K

Vitamin K is necessary for the normal clotting of blood. A dietary deficiency is unlikely, partly because the vitamin is widespread in vegetable foods such as spinach, cabbage and cauliflower, peas and cereals, and partly because our intestinal bacteria can synthesize it.

9 Recommended intakes of nutrients

An adequate intake of all the nutrients is essential for health and activity, and there are additional requirements for growth, pregnancy, lactation and in times of stress such as infection. The exact amounts needed are different for each individual, and depend not only on such readily quantifiable factors as height, weight and sex, but also on physical activity throughout the day, the rate of internal activities such as heart beat, and the climate.

As these *requirements* can only be determined after lengthy experimentation, it is impracticable if not impossible to discuss what they are. Instead, a number of national and international bodies have *recommended* certain nutrient intakes for various groups of the population in question. These recommendations are designed to ensure that the needs of almost all healthy persons will be covered.

It follows that recommended intakes will always be higher than estimates of average requirements (except for energy and the energy-yielding constituents, which are discussed below). Conversely, the actual nutrient requirements of almost all individuals will be less than the recommended intakes. Therefore, if a person's diet consistently contains more of a nutrient than is recommended he is almost certainly obtaining more than his requirement, but if it consistently contains less he may still be obtaining enough. But the further his intake falls below the recommendations, the greater his likelihood of malnourishment with its accompanying clinical symptoms.

Energy is different from other nutrients in that appetite normally controls the intake and keeps it close to requirements, and in that intakes in excess of requirements are undesirable and may lead to obesity. The recommendation for each *group* of people is therefore set at its estimated average requirement; about half of the *individuals* in the group will thus require more and half of them will require less than this.

Table 24 summarises the daily intakes of energy, protein, two minerals and six vitamins which were recommended by the Department of Health and Social Security in a report published in 1979. They are believed to be sensible and practical for the United Kingdom, but like all such recommendations, will need to be revised in the light of new knowledge. No specific recommendations were made about any of the other nutrients, but it is probable that requirements for them will be more than met if a good mixed diet is eaten in amounts which satisfy the needs for the major nutrients. Nevertheless, the National Research Council of the United States

Table 24. **Recommended daily amounts of nutrients for population groups (Department of Health and Social Security, 1979)**

Age ranges	Energy		Protein	Calcium	Iron
years	MJ	kcal	g	mg	mg
Boys					
Under 1	3.25	780	19	600	6
1	5.0	1,200	30	600	7
2	5.75	1,400	35	600	7
3-4	6.5	1,560	39	600	8
5-6	7.25	1,740	43	600	10
7-8	8.25	1,980	49	600	10
9-11	9.5	2,280	56	700	12
12-14	11.0	2,640	66	700	12
15-17	12.0	2,880	72	600	12
Girls					
Under 1	3.0	720	18	600	6
1	4.5	1,100	27	600	7
2	5.5	1,300	32	600	7
3-4	6.25	1,500	37	600	8
5-6	7.0	1,680	42	600	10
7-8	8.0	1,900	48	600	10
9-11	8.5	2,050	51	700	12[2]
12-14	9.0	2,150	53	700	12[2]
15-17	9.0	2,150	53	600	12[2]
Men					
18-34 { Sedentary	10.5	2,510	62	500	10
18-34 { Moderately active	12.0	2,900	72	500	10
18-34 { Very active	14.0	3,350	84	500	10
35-64 { Sedentary	10.0	2,400	60	500	10
35-64 { Moderately active	11.5	2,750	69	500	10
35-64 { Very active	14.0	3,350	84	500	10
65-74	10.0	2,400	60	500	10
75 and over	9.0	2,150	54	500	10
Women					
18-54 { Most occupations	9.0	2,150	54	500	12[2]
18-54 { Very active	10.5	2,500	62	500	12[2]
55-74	8.0	1,900	47	500	10
75 and over	7.0	1,680	42	500	10
Pregnant	10.0	2,400	60	1,200	13
Lactating	11.5	2,750	69	1,200	15

[1] Most people who go out in the sun need no dietary source of vitamin D (p. 51), but children and adolescen in winter, and housebound adults, are recommended to take 10 μg vitamin D daily.
[2] These iron recommendations may not cover heavy menstrual losses.

| Vitamin A (retinol equivalent) | Thiamin | Riboflavin | Niacin equivalent | Vitamin C | Vitamin D[1] |
	mg	mg	mg	mg	μg
₊50	0.3	0.4	5	20	7.5
₆00	0.5	0.6	7	20	10
₆00	0.6	0.7	8	20	10
₆00	0.6	0.8	9	20	10
₆00	0.7	0.9	10	20	–
₆00	0.8	1.0	11	20	–
₆75	0.9	1.2	14	25	–
₇25	1.1	1.4	16	25	–
₇50	1.2	1.7	19	30	–
₄50	0.3	0.4	5	20	7.5
₆00	0.4	0.6	7	20	10
₆00	0.5	0.7	8	20	10
₆00	0.6	0.8	9	20	10
₆00	0.7	0.9	10	20	–
₆00	0.8	1.0	11	20	–
₆75	0.8	1.2	14	25	–
₇25	0.9	1.4	16	25	–
₇50	0.9	1.7	19	30	–
₇50	1.0	1.6	18	30	–
₇50	1.2	1.6	18	30	–
₇50	1.3	1.6	18	30	–
₇50	1.0	1.6	18	30	–
₇50	1.1	1.6	18	30	–
₇50	1.3	1.6	18	30	–
₇50	1.0	1.6	18	30	–
₇50	0.9	1.6	18	30	–
₇50	0.9	1.3	15	30	–
₇50	1.0	1.3	15	30	–
₇50	0.8	1.3	15	30	–
₇50	0.7	1.3	15	30	–
₇50	1.0	1.6	18	60	10
₂00	1.1	1.8	21	60	10

has made specific recommendations for folic acid, vitamin B_6, vitamin B_{12}, vitamin E, magnesium, zinc, phosphorus and iodine in the 1980 edition of their 'Recommended Dietary Allowances'. It has also estimated the daily intakes of pantothenic acid, biotin, vitamin K, sodium, potassium, chloride, copper, chromium, fluoride, manganese, molybdenum and selenium which should be both adequate and safe for health.

Some further points to be borne in mind are:

Energy The recommendations in Table 24 were based on the energy intake or expenditure of groups of the UK population, and refer to average or reference weights. Although there is normally no need for adjustment for groups of different weights, there is evidence that average energy intakes are now lower, perhaps in relation to our reduced energy expenditure.

The average values for infants under one year conceals the rapid growth which occurs during this time. The daily intakes recommended during the first year are:

	Boys			Girls		
	Energy		Protein	Energy		Protein
	kcal	MJ	g	kcal	MJ	g
Birth to 3 months	530	2.2	13	500	2.1	12.5
3 up to 6 months	720	3.0	18	670	2.8	17
6 up to 9 months	880	3.7	22	810	3.4	20
9 up to 12 months	980	4.1	24.5	910	3.8	23

Protein The intakes recommended for the UK are somewhat arbitrary, and represent 10 per cent of the energy requirement (e.g., for pregnant women, the 60 g protein recommended provides, at 4 kcal per gram, 240 kcal; this is 10 per cent of the recommended energy intake of 2400 kcal). This level ensures a palatable diet and adequate provision of nutrients which tend to accompany protein in foods, but man can consume much smaller quantities of protein and still retain good health. It should, however, be noted that if energy requirements are not fully met at the same time, that protein which is eaten will be utilized more to provide the needed energy than for growth and tissue repair.

Fat and Carbohydrate There appears to be no absolute dietary requirement for either fat or carbohydrate, except for a small amount (1-2 per cent of energy requirements) of essential fatty acids; some carbohydrate (50-100 g/day) is also necessary to prevent the undesirable effects which result from extremely high fat diets.

However, in contrast to the recommendations for protein, minerals and vitamins, which are designed to ensure that the intakes by different groups of the population are high enough for health, a number of bodies in developed countries have suggested dietary guidelines to *restrict* intakes of fat, sugars and alcohol. This is because there is growing concern that some individuals are obtaining too much of these nutrients (and not enough dietary fibre). Such guidelines may also recommend limiting intakes of salt or sodium. In the UK the Department of Health and Social Security has recommended limits on fat and saturated – plus – *trans* fatty acids (page 13), but there are no specific recommendations as to the amounts of sugars, starches or dietary fibre to be eaten by men, women or children in this country.

Calcium and Iron Both recommendations allow for the limited absorption of these nutrients from the diet.

Niacin and Vitamin A The intakes recommended allow for the likely contributions made by tryptophan and carotenes to the pre-formed nicotinic acid and retinol intakes respectively.

Vitamin C There are differing opinions as to the quantity of vitamin C required for health. It is generally agreed that 10 mg daily will not only prevent but also cure scurvy. The recommended intake of 30 mg is thought to provide a reasonable safety margin; there is no nutritional advantage from enormously higher intakes although there may be some pharmacological action.

Vitamin D It is not possible to make firm estimates of dietary needs because most of our requirements are met by vitamin D formed from the action of sunlight on a substance present in the skin. The amounts recommended may be considered as a safety measure for those who are little exposed to sunlight.

Excessive intakes of many of the minerals can be harmful, as can excessive intakes of some of the vitamins – especially vitamins A and D which accumulate in the liver. Such intakes are unlikely to arise from food, but may result from the over-enthusiastic use of mineral and vitamin supplements. Although our storage capacity for most nutrients apart from energy (as fat) is limited, the healthy body nevertheless contains enough reserves to last for many weeks or months even when there is *none* in the diet. Thus, while recommended intakes are most conveniently expressed in daily terms, it is not necessary for the diet to contain these quantities *every* day. It is sufficient if the requirements are met over a period of, say, a week.

PART 2

Nutritional value of food and diets

10 Introduction, and general effects of preparation and processing

Introduction

This part of the manual discusses the nutritional importance of particular foods in the context of the diet as a whole.

The nutritional importance of any food depends upon:

(a) The composition of the raw food or ingredients as grown or purchased

(b) The extent to which its nutrients are lost during storage, preparation or cooking, and any addition of nutrients during manufacture

(c) The amount that is usually eaten

(d) Each individual's own nutritional needs and the extent to which they have already been met by other foods in the diet.

Many factors combine to produce variations in the nutrient content of foods. *Representative* values for the most important nutrients in a wide selection of foods are given in tables throughout this manual and in Appendix 2 (page 105), and these should constantly be referred to when using this part of the book. It must be remembered, however, that individual samples or brands may differ considerably from the values quoted. A wider selection of foods and nutrients can be found in the textbook *The Composition of Foods* (1978), and in its supplement on *Immigrant Foods* (1985) as described on page 125, for those who wish to estimate their nutrient intakes in more detail.

The general effects of storage, preparation and cooking are discussed below, and the application of these principles to specific foods and menus is described in Chapters 11 and 12.

Average nutrient intakes in Britain, and the contributions made by major types of food, are shown in Table 25. This table is derived from the National Food Survey, which is a long-running survey conducted by the Ministry of Agriculture, Fisheries and Food and includes about 8,000 representative households throughout Britain each year. Although any individual's diet and nutrient intake may depart considerably from this, much greater departures are likely to occur in other countries where the general dietary pattern can be quite different from those in this country.

Table 25. Percentage contributions made by groups of foods to the nutrient content of the average household diet

	Energy	Protein	Fat	Carbo-hydrate	Dietary fibre	Calcium	Iron	Sodium	Vitamin A (retinol equivalent)	Thiamin	Vitamin C
Milk	10	15	12	6	0	37	2	2	14	9	4
Milk products	4	7	7	1	0	19	1	4	5	2	1
TOTAL MILK, CREAM, CHEESE, ETC.	14	22	19	7	0	56	3	6	19	11	5
Carcase meat	6	13	11	0	0	0	12	1	0	5	0
Bacon and ham	2	3	4	0	0	0	1	6	0	3	0
Poultry	1	5	1	0	0	0	2	0	0	1	0
Other meat & meat products	7	10	10	2	0	3	7	8	30	5	2
TOTAL MEAT	16	31	26	2	0	3	22	15	30	14	2
FISH	1	5	1	0	0	2	2	2	0	1	0
EGGS	2	5	3	0	0	2	5	1	4	2	0
Margarine	6	0	13	0	0	0	0	3	11	0	0
Butter	5	0	11	0	0	0	1	4	8	0	0
Other oils & fats	5	0	12	0	0	0	0	0	1	0	0
TOTAL FATS	16	0	36	0	0	0	1	7	20	0	0
SUGARS & PRESERVES	8	0	0	19	0	0	1	1	0	0	1
Potatoes	5	3	0	10	16	1	6	0	0	9	19
Green vegetables	1	2	0	0	9	2	3	0	2	3	10
Root vegetables	0	0	0	4	4	1	1	0	16	1	2
Other veg & veg products	3	4	2	4	13	3	8	9	6	4	16
TOTAL VEGETABLES	9	9	2	15	42	7	18	10	24	18	47
Fresh fruit	1	0	0	3	7	1	1	0	0	2	20
Fruit products & nuts	2	1	1	3	3	1	3	0	1	2	24
TOTAL FRUIT	3	1	1	6	10	2	4	0	1	4	44
Bread and flour	17	18	3	30	33	19	23	17	0	29	0
Cakes, pastries, biscuits, & other cereal products	12	7	7	18	15	7	17	7	1	19	0
TOTAL CEREALS	29	25	10	48	48	26	40	24	1	48	0
BEVERAGES & OTHER FOODS[1]	2	2	2	3	0	2	4	34[2]	1	3	1
TOTALS	100	100	100	100	100	100	100	100	100	100	100

[1] Excluding alcoholic and soft drinks, and sweets.
[2] Mainly from salt.

Cooking and preservation

Most foods have to be prepared and cooked before they can be eaten. For some foods the process may be simple, as in the peeling of an orange. For others it may be complicated: for example wheat grains must be separated from the inedible parts of the plant and milled into flour, which in turn may need to be treated before being baked into bread. At each stage some of the nutrients will be discarded or destroyed, whether the process takes place in a factory or in the home. The nutrients may be further reduced if the food is stored for long periods, particularly if conditions are not ideal.

Although these losses are usually not of major significance if a good mixed diet is eaten (as this will still provide a considerable excess of nutrients over the recommended intakes) it is nevertheless desirable that the losses are kept to a minimum. A discussion of the main methods of cooking and preserving foods is therefore followed by descriptions of the factors which tend to reduce the stability of each nutrient. Applications to specific foods are discussed in Chapter 11.

Home cooking

Heat is generally applied to food in one of three ways:

(a) Directly, with or without additional fat – as in roasting, grilling and baking (250-475°F; 120-250°C), and microwave cooking.

(b) With water – as in boiling, stewing and braising (212°F; 100°C).

(c) With fat – frying (310-435°F; 155-225°C).

Heat causes chemical and physical changes in food which in general make the flavour, palatability and digestibility of the raw product more acceptable and may improve its keeping quality. Heat may also increase the availability of some nutrients by destroying enzymes and anti-digestive factors. But cooking more usually results in the loss of nutrients, this being greatest at high temperatures, with long cooking times, or if an excessive amount of liquid is used. The losses of soluble vitamins and minerals are, of course, reduced if meat juices and cooking water are not discarded but used in (for example) gravies.

The effects of microwaves and infra-red cooking on nutrients are similar to the effects of the more traditional methods they replace. When used for re-heating, they cause little additional destruction of nutrients.

Home freezing

This popular method of food preservation may result in some loss of thiamin and vitamin C when vegetables are blanched in water before freezing, but less than would otherwise result from the continuing action of enzymes in the plant tissues during storage. If the temperature of the freezer is kept below − 18°C (0°F) there is almost no further loss of nutritional value until the food is thawed. In general, differences between the nutrient content of cooked fresh foods and cooked frozen foods as served on the plate are small.

Industrial processing

Processing in a factory is mainly intended to preserve food so that the choice is greater and independent of geographical area or the season of the year, and to reduce the time spent on preparing food in the home. The main commercial processes which cause some loss of nutrients are blanching, heat processing, and drying or dehydration. The *freezing* process itself has little effect on nutritional value, and since the delay after harvesting is minimal the nutrients in the high quality fresh foods that are used are generally well retained. *Blanching* or scalding in water or steam is mainly to minimize enzyme activity, and is a first step in the preservation of most vegetables for subsequent canning, freezing or dehydration. The process is carefully controlled, but small amounts of some minerals and water soluble vitamins dissolve in the water or steam and are lost.

Heat processing in metal cans or bottling in glass jars will reduce the amounts of heat-sensitive vitamins, especially thiamin, folic acid and vitamin C. The losses will depend on the length of time needed to destroy any harmful organisms and to cook the food, and will be greater for larger cans and in foods of a close consistency, such as ham, because of the slow transfer of heat from the outside to the centre. They will also depend on the acidity of the food and the presence of light and air; it is therefore difficult to give precise values for expected losses.

Dehydration (in air) in carefully controlled conditions has little effect on most nutrients, but about half the vitamin C is lost and there is a complete loss of thiamin if sulphur dioxide is added as a preservative. Prolonged sun drying as in the production of raisins allows substantial changes to occur. Suitable packaging of dried foods is essential to prevent nutrient losses during their prolonged storage life.

Stability of individual nutrients

Protein is denatured by heat, and when cooking conditions are severe it will become less available for utilization within the body. This is partly because the changes in structure make the protein less readily digested and partly because some of the component amino acids will be destroyed – most notably lysine, which can react with carbohydrates in the food. These losses can also occur during prolonged storage even at room temperature.

Vitamin A Both retinol and β-carotene are stable to most cooking procedures, although at high temperatures and in the presence of air (e.g., when butter or margarine are used in frying) there will be some loss. Some loss also occurs in prolonged storage if light and air are not rigorously excluded.

The *B-vitamins* are all water soluble and most are also sensitive to heat.

Thiamin is one of the least stable of vitamins. It is readily dissolved out of foods into the cooking water and will be lost in the juices from meat. It is fairly stable to heat if the food is acid, but the losses can be considerable under alkaline conditions, for example if sodium bicarbonate is added during cooking. It has been calculated that on average about 20 per cent of the thiamin content of all the food brought into the home is lost during cooking and reheating, but the loss is greater in some foods than in others. Any foods which have been preserved by the use of sulphur dioxide, such as sausages, wine and some potato products, will contain very little thiamin.

Riboflavin will be lost in discarded cooking water and meat drippings; it is also unstable to alkali, and especially sensitive to light.

Niacin is an exceptionally stable vitamin, and will be lost only through its solubility in water.

Other B-vitamins All are soluble in water. Vitamin B_6, folic acid and panthothenic acid are also sensitive to heat, and can therefore be lost in cooking and canning.

Vitamin C is perhaps the least stable of all the vitamins. In addition to being water-soluble, it is very readily destroyed by air. This destruction is accelerated by heat, by alkali, and by the presence of certain metals, e.g., copper or iron. Vitamin C is also rapidly oxidized when an enzyme present in fruit and vegetables is released by any physical damage to the plant such as cutting. Thus poor cooking practices such as prolonged boiling of green vegetables in large amounts of water containing sodium bicarbonate to improve the colour, followed by keeping hot, can result in destruction of all the vitamin C originally present. Vitamin C is, however, partly protected by sulphur dioxide.

Vitamin D is stable to normal cooking procedures.

Vitamin E is not soluble in water and is stable to heat. It is, however, oxidized in the presence of air.

Table 26 summarizes the sensitivity of the most important nutrients.

Table 26. **Summary of factors (✓) which may reduce the nutrients in food**

Nutrient	Heat	Light	Air	Water (by leaching)	Acid	Alkali	Other
Protein	✓ if prolonged						
Minerals				✓			
Vitamin A	✓ with air		✓ with heat				Metals
Thiamin[1]	✓		✓	✓		✓	Sulphur dioxide
Riboflavin		✓		✓		✓	
Folic acid	✓		✓ (but protected by vitamin C)	✓		✓	
Vitamin C[1]	✓		✓ (but protected by sulphur dioxide)	✓		✓	Enzymes; metals

[1] Least stable to cooking and storage.

11 Foods

Milk

Importance in the diet

Cows' milk is the most complete of all foods, containing nearly all the constituents of nutritional importance to man; it is however comparatively deficient in iron and vitamins C and D. Unlike other foods of animal origin, milk contains a significant amount of carbohydrate, in the form of the disaccharide lactose (page 6).

Typical amounts of the major nutrients present in 1 pint of whole milk and of skimmed and 'semi-skimmed' milks are given below. Milk from the Jersey and Guernsey breeds of cows contains rather more fat (1 pint providing 26.7 g) as well as more β-carotene and most other vitamins and minerals.

Nutrients per pint

	Whole	Semi-skimmed	Skimmed
Energy kcal	380	267	187
kJ	1,594	1,122	796
Protein g	18.9	19.5	19.8
Fat g	22.8	9.7	0.6
Carbohydrate g	26.8	27.0	27.3
Calcium mg	604	621	633
Iron mg	0.3	0.3	0.3
Sodium mg	293	299	305
Vitamin A (retinol equivalent) μg	330	140	9
Thiamin mg	0.26	0.27	0.28
Riboflavin mg	1.01	1.04	1.05
Niacin equivalent mg	5.0	5.1	5.2
Vitamin B_{12} μg	2.5	2.5	2.6
Vitamin C mg	9[1]	9[1]	9[1]
Vitamin D μg	0.17	0.07	0

[1] Values decline on storage in the home.

Average milk consumption is now about half a pint per day, of which an increasing proportion consists of skimmed or semi-skimmed products. The contribution which these make to the nutrient content of the average household diet is shown on page 64. It can be seen that in a mixed diet milk is particularly valuable for its content of high quality protein and easily assimilated calcium, and as a rich source of riboflavin; moreover, milk provides good nutritional value for money (page 92).

Whole milk can also be a good source of energy, which is particularly important for young children. Skimmed or semi-skimmed milks may, however, be useful for those who drink a lot of milk and who wish to reduce their fat intake (page 94).

It is important that bottled milks are not left on the doorstep exposed directly to sunlight for much more than an hour, since a substantial amount of the riboflavin and vitamin C can be destroyed.

Effects of cooking

The bubbles of steam formed as milk is heated are stabilized by the protein, which causes the characteristic 'boiling over'. Food such as fish or vegetables, when baked in the milk, can cause coagulation of milk proteins, but this does not affect their digestibility. Some caramelization of the sugars in milk may occur with long cooking in a very slow oven, as for example in milk puddings or in the production of sterilized or evaporated milk.

Effects of processing

When milk is *homogenized* the fat globules are broken up mechanically and distributed throughout the milk so that they no longer rise to form a creamy layer at the top of the milk bottle. The nutritional value of homogenized milk is similar to that of pasteurized milk.

Skimmed milk has almost all of its fat removed, and *semi-skimmed* milk must by law contain only between 1.5 and 1.8 per cent fat. The fat-soluble vitamins A and D are reduced proportionately. In many products based on reduced fat milk, vitamins A and D are added by the manufacturers who may also choose to add skimmed milk powder to improve the taste. The values on page 69 are for unfortified products. *Dried skimmed milk*, and similar products with added vegetable fat, may also be fortified with vitamins A and D.

A variety of heat treatments can be used to improve the keeping quality of liquid milk. The fat, fat-soluble vitamins, carbohydrates and minerals of milk are not affected by heat – but where the heat treatment is relatively harsh, slight changes occur in the availability of some of the amino acids in the milk proteins. The vitamins in milk which are partially destroyed by heat processing are vitamin C, thiamin, pyridoxine, vitamin B_{12}, and folic acid.

Most of the liquid milk supply in Great Britain is *pasteurized*. During this mild form of heat treatment the milk is heated to about 72°C (162°F) for 15 seconds, killing any disease-causing bacteria. About 10 per cent of the thiamin and vitamin B_{12}, and 25 per cent of the vitamin C are destroyed, but in a mixed diet milk is not an important source of these nutrients. Very similar losses occur when milk is *spray dried*. The ultra-high temperature

(UHT) treatment of milk, in which a temperature of about 130°C (266°F) is maintained for one or two seconds, also causes some vitamin losses which are very similar to the losses in pasteurization. UHT or 'long-life' milk is packed aseptically into special containers which protect it from light and from oxygen. It will keep satisfactorily for several months without refrigeration, but variable losses of vitamin C and folic acid may occur during prolonged storage. Once opened, however, UHT milk is as perishable as fresh milk.

Sterilized milk is subjected to a more drastic form of heat treatment; it is prepared from homogenized milk which is bottled and then heated to about 120°C (248°F) for 20-60 minutes. About 60 per cent of the vitamin C in the raw milk and 20 per cent of the thiamin are destroyed during the process.

Evaporated milk is prepared by the concentration of liquid milk at low temperatures; the milk is subsequently sterilized in cans at 115°C (239°F) for 15 minutes. In general, the nutrient losses are similar to those in sterilized milk.

Sweetened condensed milk is prepared similarly, but since it contains added sucrose the processing temperature needed for an adequate storage life is lower. Nutrient losses are therefore lower too, and are generally similar to those that occur in pasteurization.

Milk products

Cream

Cream is derived from fresh milk either by skimming off the fatty layer which rises to the surface or in a mechanical separator. Minimum fat contents for different types of cream are specified in Government Regulations; these include: half cream, 12 per cent by weight as milk fat; single cream, 18 per cent; whipping cream 35 per cent; double cream 48 per cent; and clotted cream, 55 per cent fat. These compare with an average of 3.9 per cent fat in milk. The energy value of different types of cream varies directly with the fat content.

Yogurt

The nutritional value of yogurt is similar to that of the milk and minor ingredients used in its preparation, except that in products with added sugar or added fat the energy content is increased. Most commercial yogurts are based either on whole milk or on skimmed milk which is inoculated with a selected culture of lactic bacteria under controlled conditions. Dried skimmed milk may be added to produce a firmer consistency; flavourings, fruit juices, fruit, nuts and sugar are often incorporated to give a varied product. Some varieties of yogurt are fortified with vitamins A and D.

71

Butter

Butter is made by churning cream in a rotating drum so that the fat globules separate from the liquid buttermilk. In this country butter must contain not less than 78-80 per cent milk fat and not more than 16 per cent water. 1-2 per cent of salt is added to salted butter during manufacture. The amounts of vitamins A and D in butter are variable; representative values are shown in Appendix 2. **Margarine** is not a dairy product but a butter substitute made by homogenizing a mixture of oils and fats with brine. Almost any edible oils can be used for margarine and for the low-fat spreads which contain about 40 per cent fat, as their physical properties can be modified first to give different proportions of the various fatty acids (page 11). Vitamins A and D must by law be added to margarine for retail sale. The values required are 760 to 940 international units of vitamin A and 80 to 100 international units of vitamin D per ounce, which are equivalent to 800-1,000 micrograms retinol and 7-9 micrograms vitamin D per 100 grams. **Ghee** is made by the prolonged heating of butter. The emulsion breaks down and on cooling the pure fat can be separated from the water. Vegetable ghee can also be obtained.

Cheese

When rennet is added to warm acidified milk, the milk protein casein coagulates to form a firm curd which is treated in various ways to make cheeses of different kinds. Most of the protein, fat and vitamin A and much of the calcium in the milk remain in the curd, while a large part of the lactose and B-vitamins are lost with the whey as it drains away. Further minor changes in vitamin content occur during ripening and storage, processes which are greatly affected by the amount of salt present. Cheddar cheese consists very roughly of one-third protein, one-third fat and one-third water; although methods of preparation differ, the amounts of protein, fat and carbohydrate in whole milk cheeses are fairly similar. *Cottage cheese* is made from skimmed milk and therefore contains very little fat; *cream cheese* has a high fat content. Hard cheeses such as Cheddar and double Gloucester in general contain more nutrients per 100 grams than soft cheeses such as Camembert because they contain less moisture. Certain cheeses are made from milk other than cows' milk; for example feta cheese is made from goats' or sheep's milk.

Ice cream

The nutrient composition of dairy **ice cream** varies with the amounts of sugar, milk, dried milk, butterfat and cream which it contains; it can make a useful contribution to the daily intake of energy and calcium, particularly for people who have small appetites or who will not drink milk. However, most ice cream is based on skimmed milk with non-dairy fats instead of or as well as milk fat.

Eggs

Importance in the diet

Eggs make a useful contribution to the daily intake of vitamin D, retinol, riboflavin, iodine, iron and protein in the average diet and for the elderly they can be a particularly important source of protein, iron, vitamin B_{12} and vitamin D. The extent to which the iron is absorbed is dependent on the other components of the meal; it has been shown for example, that the addition of orange juice increases its absorption.

The shell colour is related to the breed of hen rather than to nutrient content and in this respect it is therefore unimportant; similarly a deep yellow yolk does not necessarily indicate a high vitamin A content since the pigment is not β-carotene.

It has been shown that there is no practical difference in the composition of eggs obtained from battery, deep litter and free range hens.

Effects of cooking

When eggs are boiled or fried the proteins coagulate first in the white at approximately 60°C (140°F), then in the yolk. This property of coagulation makes eggs suitable for binding dry ingredients together in cooking, and for thickening sauces and soups; the mixture of eggs and milk sets in baked egg custard. Over-cooking causes the proteins to curdle and contract slightly and a yellow watery fluid separates out; this may occur when scrambling eggs or boiling sauces to which eggs have been added.

The black discoloration which is sometimes present around the yolk of hard boiled eggs is iron sulphide which is formed during cooking from hydrogen sulphide in the egg white and iron in the egg yolk; this blackening can be reduced by cooling the eggs in water immediately after cooking. When egg whites are beaten, the proteins will hold air and form a stable foam which coagulates or sets at a very low temperature, as for example in meringues. Eggs are also used as raising agents, e.g., in sponge cakes, and to promote the emulsification of fat, e.g., in mayonnaise. Some of the heat-sensitive B-vitamins are lost during cooking. For example, the average loss of thiamin which results from boiling, frying, poaching and scrambling is between 5 and 15 per cent; similar losses of riboflavin also occur. During frying, the fat content of eggs may be increased by about 50 per cent.

Meat

The average nutrient composition of various types of meat is shown in Appendix 2. Changes in methods of animal husbandry have led to the introduction of new breeds and the slaughter of younger animals; the meat is therefore more tender and has less fat than before, and its flavour tends to be less pronounced. More of the external fat is also trimmed off prior to sale.

Muscle tissue is composed of bundles of muscle fibres surrounded by connective tissue and associated with intramuscular fat. Each separate muscle fibre is a tube composed largely of water, and containing soluble proteins, mineral salts, vitamins and flavours. The eating quality of meat is largely determined by the relative proportions of connective tissue and muscle fibres in a particular cut and the amount of 'marbling' fat that is present within the lean, but the overall nutrient content of *lean* meat from the more expensive cuts is not significantly different from that in other parts of the carcase.

Importance in the diet

Meat is a good source of high quality protein, of available iron and zinc, and of all the B-vitamins except folic acid. Pork, bacon and ham in particular are rich in thiamin. Liver and to a lesser extent kidney, are also rich in vitamin A and folic acid (thus differing from carcase meat) and in iron, riboflavin and other B-vitamins. Sweetbreads and tripe are useful and easily digestible sources of animal protein. Tripe also contains more calcium than other meats; this is derived from the lime with which it is treated during preparation. Chicken, turkey, liver and kidney contain less fat than most carcase meat and their energy content is therefore lower. Much of the fat can nevertheless be trimmed from beef, lamb and pork before or after cooking.

Consumption of poultry meat is twelve times greater than in 1955; this trend is due to the growth of the broiler industry and the consequent fall in the price of poultry. Small differences in the nutrient composition of broiler chickens and free range chickens are of no significance in a mixed diet.

Effects of cooking

The muscle protein myoglobin which provides the red colour of raw meat is changed by heat, and the brown colour associated with cooked meat develops at temperatures above 65°C. Heat causes the proteins in the muscle fibres to coagulate and the meat becomes firm: shrinkage occurs and this in turn causes extrusion of meat juices and a loss of weight. Losses of fat and meat juices increase as the temperature rises, so the total weight loss is influenced by the cooking temperature and the internal temperature to which the meat is cooked as well as by the cooking time: thus the effects of grilling and frying are similar. The substantial variations that occur in the proportions of bone, muscle and fat in different parts of different carcases also affect the nutrients that are actually available from a given weight of fresh meat. It is thus very important, when estimating the contributions made by meat to the nutrient content of a diet, to weigh each cut *after* cooking and removal of any fat or bone.

Some cheaper cuts of meat which contain a higher proportion of connective tissue are more palatable if a slow moist method of cooking, such as stewing or braising, is used for their preparation; this allows the collagen in the connective tissue to be converted to gelatin thus making the meat more tender. Pressure cooking is also useful for this purpose.

Cooking does not affect the minerals present in meat but a proportion of those which are soluble pass into the drip or dissolve in the cooking water. Similarly, since the B-vitamins are all water-soluble, varying amounts will be found in the drip, meat juice or stock. Cooking temperatures have relatively little effect on niacin or riboflavin; thiamin, pyridoxine, folic acid and pantothenic acid are more sensitive to heat, and destruction varies between 30 and 50 per cent. After cooking, there are only small differences in the content of the B-vitamins in fresh and frozen meat. Vitamin A is relatively stable to heat, and is not affected by most cooking procedures, although some loss occurs during frying at high temperatures (above 200°C).

There is no evidence of any significant loss of nutrients from meat during *freezing*, but the drip which collects on thawing will contain some soluble nutrients.

Meat extractives are water-soluble substances from meat which include peptides, B-vitamins and mineral salts; they provide, with fat, most of the flavour and aroma of meat and act as a stimulant to appetite and to the secretion of gastric juice.

Stock can be made by boiling meat bones in water. The hot water extracts a small amount of fat and gelatin from the bone marrow together with other minor components which provide the flavour. Stock is usually used as a basis for soup and it is the addition of other ingredients, e.g., milk, fat and flour in cream soups, which provides most of the nutritional value of the soup.

Meat products

The meat content of meat products such as sausages is controlled by Regulations (page 122). The important contribution which they make to the nutrient content of the average household diet is shown on page 64; average consumption per head is now rather greater than for carcase meat.

The most usual methods of *heat treatment* before any domestic cooking are smoking and canning, both of which cause some loss of thiamin and a slight reduction in the quality of the meat protein. The loss of thiamin when meat is canned is generally slightly greater than in cooked meat. Corned beef is prepared from cured meat which is trimmed, coarsely cut and cooked before canning; after this process very little thiamin remains in the finished product. Commercial *meat extract* is a by-product of corned beef manufacture. The liquid in which successive batches of meat have been heated is concentrated after the removal of the fat. Such products, including stock cubes, are also rich in salt. When the meat extract containing the dissolved solids is diluted again for consumption, the amount of protein and energy which it contributes to the soup or beverage is too small to be of importance in the diet; nevertheless it contains minerals besides the salt and vitamins, and is a useful stimulant to appetite.

The nutrient losses that occur during the cooking of meat products are similar to those on cooking carcase meat.

Fish

Importance in the diet

The flesh or muscle of fish is a valuable source of protein which is of a similar quality to that of meat and milk. It can be seen from Appendix 2 that the amount of fat in different kinds of fish varies widely; the flesh of white fish, such as cod, haddock, plaice and whiting, contains very little fat (1-2 per cent) while that of fatty fish (herring, mackerel, trout, salmon, eel) varies from 10 per cent to more than 20 per cent. In general, the vitamin content of white fish muscle is similar to that of lean meat. The fat-soluble vitamins A and D are present in the flesh of fatty fish and in the livers of fish such as cod and halibut; oils from the latter may therefore be used as concentrated vitamin supplements. Fish muscle also contains a well balanced supply of minerals including iodine, and if the bones are eaten, as for example in sardines and canned salmon, these are a good source of calcium, phosphorus and fluoride.

Effects of cooking and processing

The changes that occur when fish is cooked are similar to those in meat but the shrinkage is not so great; losses of mineral salts are proportional to the loss of water. The vitamin A and vitamin D in fatty fish are both heat stable. When fish is canned or cured by smoking there is some loss of thiamin, but otherwise these processes have little effect on the nutrients in fish. Modern methods of freezing do not affect the nutritive value. For estimating the cooked weight of fish, a loss of about 15 per cent may be assumed on gentle cooking unless frying is used: fish fried in batter and fried fish products will gain fat on cooking.

Sugars and preserves

White sugar provides energy and no other nutrient. Brown sugars and honey also include insignificant quantities of minerals and some B-vitamins, but nowhere near enough of the latter to assist with the metabolism of the sugars present (page 44). Some preserves contain vitamin C and chocolate contains iron and other nutrients, but the main function of all these foods in the diet is to increase palatability.

Vegetables

Importance in the diet

Notwithstanding the fact that they contain 80-95 per cent of water, vegetables, including potatoes, supply appreciable quantities of nutrients in the average diet and they are also an important source of dietary fibre (page 8). The low energy content, bulky nature and range of colours of many vegetables (and fruits) are responsible for their extensive use in the many attractive and appetizing meals which are frequently recommended to 'slimmers' (page 96). The composition of different vegetables is given in Appendix 2; their nutrient content is influenced by a number of factors during growth and after harvesting and different samples of the same vegetable can vary considerably. For example, the amount of vitamin C will vary with variety, maturity and exposure to sunlight, as well as with the method of handling, the temperature during transport and the delay before the 'fresh' product is eaten.

Green vegetables

These are of nutritional importance because of their contribution to the daily intake of vitamin C, β-carotene (which after absorption is converted to vitamin A in the body), folic acid, iron and other minerals, and dietary fibre. They are especially valuable when eaten raw, as they will suffer no cooking losses; there will be, however, considerable losses of vitamin C in wilted vegetables.

Potatoes

In many diets potatoes provide the main source of vitamin C, even though the vitamin content per unit weight is comparatively low. The amount is highest in new potatoes and falls gradually during post-harvest storage. Instant potato powder and potato flakes or granules are nutritionally equivalent alternatives to fresh potatoes only if the vitamin C and thiamin which are lost in processing are added back to the products. Because of the comparatively large amounts which are eaten, potatoes contribute more protein and iron than other vegetables in the average diet and they are also useful sources of thiamin, niacin and several other nutrients including dietary fibre.

Root vegetables

Nearly one quarter of the average daily intake of vitamin A is provided by vegetables, most of this (17 per cent) by carrots. In contrast, turnips, swedes and parsnips are comparatively good sources of vitamin C, but they contain no β-carotene.

Peas and beans

Peas, and the wide range of fresh, dried, canned and frozen beans now available, are rich in protein and provide more energy, B-vitamins and dietary fibre than green and root vegetables; fresh and frozen peas and beans (but not canned processed peas, dried peas or beans, or baked beans) also contain vitamin C. It is important to remember that the apparently high levels of nutrients shown in dried peas and beans in Appendix 2 will fall when the vegetables are soaked before use.

Soya flour and other products derived from beans are increasingly being used in manufactured foods. They are nutritionally valuable, and extra nutrients may also be added if they are intended to resemble meat (see page 16).

Effects of cooking

The main purpose of cooking vegetables is to soften the cellular tissue and to gelatinize any starch that may be present so that they can be digested more easily.

Weight changes in preparation and cooking Peeling and trimming may reduce the purchased weight of some vegetables by up to one-third or more (Appendix 2); changes in the weight of most raw vegetables during boiling are small and may be ignored when making calculations from food tables.

Nutrient losses After peeling or shredding, vitamin C is rapidly destroyed by oxidation either directly or by the action of an enzyme present in the plant tissues. This loss can be kept to a minimum by preparing vegetables immediately before use, and by plunging them into boiling water (from which any dissolved oxygen will have been driven off) at the start of the cooking process, when the enzyme will be destroyed.

During cooking, nutrient losses in vegetables (and to a smaller extent in fruit) are mainly caused by the passage of soluble mineral salts and vitamins from the tissues into the cooking water, and by the destruction of some vitamins by heat. Thus, some vitamin C and thiamin are inevitably lost when water is used for cooking because they are both heat sensitive and water soluble. It follows that the greater the volume of water used, the greater is the loss. Green vegetables, which have a large surface area, lose on average between 50 and 75 per cent of their vitamin C during cooking. Average losses from potatoes are:

	per cent
Boiled after peeling	20-50
Boiled in their skins	20-40
Baked in their skins	10-40
Roasted	15-50
Chipped or fried	15-30

If cooked potatoes are mashed and then kept hot, the loss of vitamin C is greater than if they are left whole under similar conditions.

There is a further loss of vitamin C if there is a delay in service and vegetables are kept hot for any length of time. This appears to be accelerated when sodium bicarbonate has been added to the cooking water. For example, after being kept hot for 30 minutes, cabbage will provide about 60 per cent of its freshly cooked value, and after an hour, only 40 per cent of its original vitamin C.

Potato whiteners or sulphite dips prevent the discoloration of raw pre-peeled potatoes when they are prepared centrally for distribution to restaurants and other catering establishments, but the amount of thiamin which is lost when the treated potatoes are boiled or fried as chips and subsequently kept hot is greatly increased by this treatment.

The fat content of chips varies between 5 and 25 per cent of their weight. It is lowest when the chips are cut large to reduce their surface area, and when the frying oil is kept hot. The amount of the different fatty acids they or other fried vegetables contain depends on the oil or fat in which they have been fried.

It is not necessary to use salt when boiling vegetables.

Effects of processing

The general effects of processing on the nutritive value of foods are discussed on page 63.

Freezing does not in itself cause losses of vitamins, but during *canning* there is some destruction of those vitamins which are unstable to heat (see page 66).

When sulphite is added to dehydrated vegetables to preserve vitamin C and prevent deterioration of quality during storage most of the thiamin is destroyed. In general, this loss is not serious because in a mixed diet the thiamin is obtained from many other foods.

Fruit

Fruit is nutritionally most important as a major source of vitamin C in the diet, but it must be remembered that the amount in different fruits varies widely and will always be rather lower after cooking. Blackcurrants are exceptionally rich, followed by strawberries and other soft fruits, oranges, grapefruit and many fruit juices (but not fruit squash). Apples, bananas, cherries and rhubarb are examples of fruits which contain much less of the vitamin and which do not in this respect compare favourably with green vegetables. Vitamin C may be added to some fruit products such as apple juice and rose hip syrup. Most fruits also contain sugars and small amounts of other vitamins and minerals.

Commercial fruit juices are made from concentrated juice and preserved by UHT treatment (page 70). They retain their vitamin C well during prolonged storage, but once the package is opened it will slowly be lost through oxidation.

Dried fruits such as currants, sultanas, raisins, dates and figs provide energy, principally in the form of sugar. Prunes and dried apricots are also useful sources of β-carotene. Dried fruits do not contain vitamin C.

Nuts and nut products such as peanut butter and some products for vegetarians are rich in fat and protein and are consequently a concentrated source of energy. They are a good source of the B-vitamins, but contain no vitamins A or C.

Cereals

Importance in the diet

Cereal grains are a major component of man's diet throughout the world. In Britain, wheat in the form of bread, flour, cakes, biscuits and pasta together with other cereals provides more than a quarter of the total energy, protein, carbohydrate and iron in the average household diet, although the iron is poorly absorbed. Cereals also make a substantial contribution to the intake of many other nutrients, particularly calcium, niacin and thiamin which are added to most flours, sodium from added salt, and dietary fibre. In general, the common cereals (wheat, oats, barley, rye, maize and rice) contain 60-75 per cent carbohydrate (starch), 7-13 per cent protein, 1-9 per cent fat, 4-8 per cent dietary fibre and approximately 12 per cent moisture in the whole grain. Advances in plant breeding have led to the development of cereal varieties which are richer in lysine; some increases in protein levels may be obtained experimentally by the appropriate use of manures and fertilizers.

Nutrient losses in milling

The distribution of nutrients within the wheat grain is not uniform. The concentration of protein, minerals and vitamins is higher in the germ and outer layers of the grain than in the inner starchy endosperm; thus when wheat is milled to produce white flour a proportion of the nutrients and dietary fibre is discarded with the bran and germ. Because of the continuing, if decreasing, preference for white flour in the British diet, those nutrients lost in the refining process which are of importance in relation to the whole diet are restored. Similar losses of minerals and vitamins occur in the milling of rice unless it is parboiled.

The composition of flour in the UK is controlled by Regulations (page 123) which require that all flours contain the following minimum quantities of two B-vitamins (thiamin and niacin) and iron which correspond to the levels occuring naturally in 80 per cent extraction flour[1]:

---

[1] The weight of flour obtained from a given weight of cleaned grain, expressed as a percentage, is known as the *extraction rate*.

	per 100 g
Iron	1.65 mg
Thiamin (vitamin B_1)	0.24 mg
Niacin	1.60 mg

White flours of about 73 per cent extraction, as now used, have to be fortified with these nutrients to bring their concentrations to the prescribed levels; wholemeal flours contain more than the specified minimum quantities. In addition calcium carbonate must be added to all flours except wholemeal and certain self-raising flours at the rate of 235-390 mg/100 g.

Wholemeal, brown and white flours

The composition of each of these flours varies, but in general wholemeal flour contains somewhat greater amounts of most minerals and several vitamins, particularly of the B group, but less calcium than the flours to which calcium is added. Wholemeal flour also contains more dietary fibre and phytic acid than brown or white flour. However, apart from the fibre content, nutritional differences between wholemeal and the fortified brown and white flours are unlikely to be of practical significance in a mixed diet.

Flours which will produce a large loaf of good quality need to contain sufficient gluten, either from 'strong' varieties of wheat or else added separately. 'Weak' wheats give flours which are more suitable for making biscuits and cakes.

Effects of cooking and processing

Cooking causes the starch granules of which cereal carbohydrate is composed to swell and gelatinize, thus making the starch digestible (page 7); it also results in a tripling (approximately) of the weight of rice and pasta on boiling as they take up water.

Thiamin is the vitamin mainly affected during the baking or processing of cereal products because it is sensitive to heat and destroyed by alkali. The amount lost therefore varies with the cooking time and the final temperature of the cooked food, and whether or not baking powder is used as for example in bread or scones. Riboflavin and niacin are more stable to heat and the loss on baking is small. Of the other unstable vitamins, folic acid is low in wheat, and vitamin C is only present if added as a flour improver before making bread. It is then destroyed on baking.

In bread-making the yeast gradually ferments the sugars which are formed from the starch in the dough, breaking them down to alcohol and then to carbon dioxide and water which are driven off, thus causing the bread to rise. When water is added to the flour in the preparation of the dough the proteins gliadin and glutenin combine to form gluten. During baking, the yeast is killed and fermentation ceases. The gluten holds the gas and then coagulates as cooking proceeds, holding the bread in shape. The average loss of thiamin in baking bread is about 15 per cent.

About 80 per cent of the bread sold in Britain is now made by the *Chorleywood Bread Process* in which conventional fermentation of the dough is replaced by a few minutes of intense mechanical agitation in special high speed mixers. This allows a greater proportion of UK wheats to be used, but it has been shown that breads produced by this process do not differ significantly in nutritional value from those made by conventional methods.

Toast

When bread is toasted the thiamin content is further reduced; the total loss on toasting varies between 15 per cent in thick slices and 30 per cent in thin slices. The heat drives off water from the bread, so that the content of energy and other nutrients per unit weight increases.

Cakes and biscuits

When making a cake, such as a Madeira cake, air is introduced into the mixture by creaming together the fat and sugar. The eggs are lightly beaten to incorporate air before adding to the creamed mixture and the flour is folded in lightly so that this air is not forced out. During cooking the starch gelatinizes and the flour and egg proteins coagulate. The loss of thiamin when making cakes and biscuits varies between 20 and 30 per cent.

The relative proportions of fat and sugar to flour and other ingredients are important in giving different cakes and biscuits their characteristic textures and tastes.

Breakfast cereals

The heat treatment used in the preparation of breakfast cereals destroys a large proportion of the thaimin present in the whole grain. In puffed and flaked products it is usually a total loss but the process used in the preparation of shredded wheat is less drastic and only about half the thiamin is destroyed. Many breakfast cereals are therefore enriched with vitamin B_1 (thiamin); protein, iron, a wide range of vitamins, sugar, salt and bran are also added to many products, which are now an important source of nutrients for many people. When porridge is made from coarse oatmeal the cooking loss of thiamin is about 10 per cent.

Alcohol

The alcohol in alcoholic drinks is rapidly absorbed from the digestive tract and utilized as a source of energy, 1 gram of alcohol providing 7 kilocalories or 29 kilojoules. Carbohydrate may also be present in varying proportions and this provides additional energy. Consumption of spirits, beer and wine continues to rise and it is estimated that in the UK more than 200 kcal

(850 kJ) per adult per day are on average obtained from alcoholic drink. Chronic alcoholics may obtain a large proportion of their energy intake from alcohol and eat very little food. Beer contains significant amounts of riboflavin and niacin, but spirits contain no vitamins; inevitably the displacement of food by alcohol leads to a marked reduction in the intake of protein, vitamins and many other nutrients.

Table 27. **Energy constituents of some alcoholic drinks, average values per 100 ml**

	Alcohol g	Carbohydrate g	Energy kcal	kJ
Beer, bitter	4.1	2.3	37	156
Lager	3.9	<0.1	29	122
Cider, sweet	3.7	4.3	95	176
Sherry, medium	16.8	5.9	140	582
Red wine	12.1	0.1	85	353
White wine, dry	9.1	0.6	66	275
White wine, sweet	10.2	5.9	94	390
Spirits	31.7	0	222	919
Liqueurs, medium strength	25.1	32.8	299	1,253

1 ml of pure alcohol weighs 0.79 g.

12 Nutritional value of meals and diets

The diet as a whole

The nutritional value of a person's diet depends upon the overall mixture of foods that is eaten during the course of weeks, months or years, and upon the needs of the individual eating them. No single food can be 'good' or 'bad' in isolation. Thus it is *consistent* overeating and not the occasional overindulgence that results in obesity; conversely, it takes a consistent reduction in energy intake or increase in energy expenditure and not sporadic bouts of starvation to effect permanent weight loss. Similarly, scurvy will not result from a diet containing little or no vitamin C for a few days, nor is there a likelihood of a heart attack from eating too much fat at one meal or from enjoying foods that are rich in fat, *unless* such practices are repeated for long periods. And even then, there is such variation in individual's needs for energy and for other nutrients that it is difficult to predict the exact effects of any particular diet on health either in the short or the long term.

It is nevertheless good nutritional practice to develop basic eating patterns that are as conducive to good health as possible. This involves eating one or more balanced meals per day (page 90), with a variety of foods chosen from among the cereals, vegetables, fruit, meat or fish, and dairy products, and a limited consumption of snacks. The diet is much more likely to contain enough vitamin C, for example, if fruit, fruit juice or vegetables are eaten every day than if they are eaten only at irregular intervals. Such guidelines are especially important for people whose needs are high and whose appetites may be small, such as young children and pregnant women.

Number of meals per day

A meal can be arbitrarily defined as the amount of food eaten at one period of time, and which provides 200 kcal (850 kJ) or more. This definition covers much more than the popular meaning of the word, which is that of hot, cooked food eaten while sitting down. People may eat from two to six or more such meals a day, the arrangement being determined mainly by custom, life style and by working conditions. Although the amounts of nutrients in different meals may vary, the total intake of each nutrient should meet an individual's needs, ideally each day and certainly over a period of a week, if the food eaten is to be fully adequate for health.

There is evidence that the number of meals taken in a day (and consequently the amount of food eaten at one time) influences the pattern of utilization of nutrients by the body.

Eating between meals

People who eat sweets or chocolates between meals or eat a large number of snacks are likely to have a reduced appetite for vegetables, cereals or meat at the next main meal. This is bad nutritional practice. Firstly, the intake of protein and other nutrients from the main meal will be reduced, and secondly, excessive consumption of sweets can result in severe dental decay. Eating high energy foods between meals, particularly those rich in fat or sugar (such as crisps and chocolate biscuits), can also result in an undesirable increase in weight if the total daily energy intake then exceeds the energy used up. For adults, alcoholic drinks are frequently a cause of excess energy intake.

Breakfast

Because of the length of time since the previous meal, and the consequent low blood sugar in the morning, it is good nutritional practice to eat breakfast before starting work. It is particularly important for children and people in demanding jobs to have a good breakfast because this helps to keep them alert during the morning. Two possible breakfasts are shown in Table 28. One is a common British breakfast, while the other has been modified to provide less fat and saturated fatty acids but more dietary fibre. Both provide adequate amounts of energy, protein and a wide range of minerals and vitamins, although the latter provides more sodium.

Calculation of nutrients in prepared dishes and meals, using food tables

Dishes

Appendix 2 gives the nutrient composition of many of the ingredients which may be used in mixed dishes. From the recipe, the approximate nutritional value of a dish can then be worked out by arithmetic. To illustrate this, the calculation of the nutritional value of a homemade cheese and tomato pizza is shown in Table 29. An allowance has been made for the change in weight and probable loss of thiamin and vitamin C during cooking.

Meals

It is not uncommon to have a choice between two types of meal: for example, one could be a cooked meal and the other a sandwich-based meal which many people might not consider to be a meal at all. Table 30 compares the nutrient

Table 28. **Comparison of two breakfasts**

	Weight g	Energy kcal	Protein g	Fat g	Saturated fatty acids g	Dietary fibre[1] g	Sodium mg
Light breakfast I							
Cornflakes	28	103	2.4	0.5	0.06	0.2/2.4	325
Sugar	10	39	0	0	0	0	0
Milk, whole	112	73	3.6	4.4	2.80	0	56
White bread (1 slice)	25	58	2.1	0.4	0.09	0.4/1.0	131
Margarine, hard	7	52	0	5.7	2.21	0	56
Marmalade	10	26	0	0	0	0	0
Milk (whole) in 2 cups tea	56	36	1.8	2.2	1.40	0	28
TOTAL		387	9.9	13.2	6.56	0.6/3.4	596
Light breakfast II							
All Bran	28	76	4.2	1.6	0.27	6.6/7.3	468
Sugar	10	39	0	0	0	0	0
Milk (semi-skimmed)	112	52	3.7	1.9	1.22	0	56
Wholemeal bread (thick slice)	54	116	4.9	1.4	0.28	4.4/4.8	302
Margarine, soft	7	52	0	5.7	1.70	0	56
Marmalade	10	26	0	0	0	0	0
Milk (semi-skimmed) in 2 cups tea	56	26	1.9	1.0	0.61	0	28
TOTAL		387	14.7	11.6	4.08	11.0/12.1	910

[1]Values depend on the method of analysis (see page 8).

Table 29. **Nutrients in a homemade cheese and tomato pizza**

Ingredient	Wt g	Energy kcal	Energy kJ	Protein g	Fat g	Carbo-hydrate g	Dietary fibre[1] g	Calcium mg	Iron mg	Sodium mg	Vitamin A (retinol equiv-alent) mg	Thiamin mg	Ribo-flavin mg	Niacin equiv-alent mg	Vitamin C mg
Flour mixture:															
White	75	253	1,076	7.1	1.0	57.5	3.0	105	1.5	1.5	0	0.233	0.030	2.63	0
Wholemeal	75	230	977	9.5	1.7	47.1	6.0	29	2.9	1.5	0	0.353	0.068	6.23	0
Baking powder	5	8	35	0.3	0	1.9	0	56	0	590	0	0	0	0	0
Margarine	50	365	753	0	20.3	0	0	2	0.1	400	450	0	0	0.05	0
Milk	75	49	204	2.4	2.9	3.5	0	77	0.1	38	42	0.038	0.128	0.68	1.1
Oil	10	90	370	0	10.0	0	0	0	0	0	0	0	0	0	0
Onion	100	23	99	0.9	0	5.2	1.3	31	0.3	10	0	0.03	0.05	0.4	10
Tomatoes, fresh	300	42	180	2.7	0	8.4	4.5	39	1.2	9	300	0.18	0.12	2.4	60
Cheddar cheese	150	609	2,523	39.0	50.3	0	0	1,200	0.6	915	545	0.06	0.75	9.3	0
Whole pizza	722[2]	1,668	6,217	61.9	86.1	123.6	14.8	1,539	6.7	1,965	1,337	0.76[3]	1.15	21.7	43[3]
Per 100 g		231	861	8.6	11.9	17.1	2.0	213	0.9	272	185	0.10	0.16	3.0	5.9

[1] Dietary fibre values will be lower if a different analytical method is used (page 8).
[2] The total weight is less than the sum of the ingredients owing to the loss of moisture in cooking.
[3] 15% of thiamin deducted to allow for loss in cooking; 40% of vitamin C deducted to allow for loss in cooking.

Table 30. Comparison of the nutritional value of a snack and a cooked meal.

	Wt g	Energy kcal	Protein g	Fat g	Carbo-hydrate g	Calcium mg	Iron mg	Sodium mg	Vitamin A µg	Thiamin mg	Ribo-flavin mg	Niacin equiv-alent mg	Vitamin C mg
Snack meal													
Bread, brown	120	260.4	10.08	2.40	53.04	118.8	2.64	648	0	0.324	0.120	2.76	0
Butter	24	177.6	0.10	19.68	0	3.6	0.05	209	236	0	0	0.02	0
Ham	56	93.0	9.18	6.22	0	2.2	0.34	787	0	0.302	0.112	3.53	0
Pickle	28	37.5	0.17	0.08	9.63	5.3	0.56	476	0	0.008	0.003	0.06	0
Banana	120	91.2	1.32	0	23.04	8.4	0.48	1	40	0.048	0.084	0.96	12
Coffee	2	2.0	0.29	0	0.22	2.8	0.09	2	0	0.001	0.004	0.56	0
Milk, whole	28	18.2	0.90	1.09	1.29	28.8	0.03	14	16	0.014	0.048	0.25	0.39
Total		679.9	22.04	29.47	87.22	169.9	4.19	2,137	292	0.697	0.371	8.14	12.39
Cooked meal													
Roast chicken (meat only)	100	148.0	24.80	5.40	0	9.0	0.80	81	0	0.080	0.190	12.80	0
Chips	110	257.4	3.96	11.22	37.4	15.4	0.92	45	0	0.220	0.022	1.65	11
Peas	84	60.5	5.04	0.76	8.99	29.4	1.34	2	42	0.252	0.076	1.34	10.08
Trifle	140	231.0	3.08	12.88	27.30	95.2	0.42	88	70	0.084	0.140	0.84	0
Total		696.9	36.88	30.26	73.69	149.0	3.48	216*	112	0.636	0.428	16.63	21.08

*Sodium from salt added at the table has not been included.

content of two ham sandwiches, a banana and coffee with that of roast chicken, chips, peas and trifle, as calculated from the figures given in Appendix 2. It can be seen that the two meals have a very similar energy value, and that this particular snack is richer than the cooked meal in calcium, iron and vitamin A although it contains less niacin and vitamin C. These sandwiches will also contain more dietary fibre, and considerably more sodium unless the cooked meal is salted during cooking or at the table.

A cold or packed meal is thus not necessarily inferior to a cooked meal: the nutritional value of both depend on the quantity and nutrient content of the items within them.

Allowance for waste

The calculation of the nutritional value of a meal or a diet *as actually eaten* cannot be made directly from the total amounts of the foods bought from the shops, nor from the total food used in the kitchen. There is always a proportion of waste for which allowance must be made, that is:
1. INEDIBLE WASTE, e.g. egg shells, potato peelings, outer leaves of cabbages, orange peel, bacon rinds, bones and gristle of meat etc.
2. EDIBLE WASTE
    (a) *Preparation losses*, e.g., batter left in mixing bowls, fat trimmed from meat or left in frying pans, crusts from bread, spilt milk.
    (b) *Table waste*, e.g., scraps left on plates.
    (c) *Pet food*, e.g., edible scraps fed to domestic pets, garden birds, ducks.
    (d) Edible food which has 'gone bad' and is discarded.

Inedible waste

Average figures for the inedible waste associated with different foods are given in Appendix 2 as a percentage of the product as listed. For example, 40 per cent of bananas (item 103), as purchased, is skin which is not eaten.

The food tables throughout this Manual always give the nutrients in the 'edible portion', and if they are used for calculating the nutritional value of foods where only the purchased weight is known the percentage of inedible waste must be deducted. For example, the energy value of one kilogram of bananas (purchased weight) will be:

$$10 \times \frac{100\text{-}40}{100} \times (\text{kcal per 100 g, from Appendix 2})$$

$$= 10 \times \frac{60}{100} \times 76$$

$$= 456 \text{ kcal}$$

Further examples of this type of calculation are given in Appendix 3.

The percentage of inedible waste in a food varies with the exact nature of the food and with its quality. For example, it varies between different cuts and joints of beef and between different sizes and varieties of orange. The values given must therefore be used with discretion.

Edible waste

It is often difficult for practical reasons to measure the weight of food actually eaten, for example by a particular individual in a large family or when a meal is eaten away from home. Estimates of portion sizes and of the loss of edible food may then need to be made before the nutritional adequacy of any diet can be worked out. The average wastage of food in the home in cooking, on plates and from food given to pets has been found to be between 5 and 10 per cent, but of course the amount varies from food to food and from family to family. Wastage can also be high in some catering establishments.

Planning balanced meals and nutritionally adequate diets

The provision of palatable and acceptable meals must be the first consideration; only within this framework can planning for good nutrition be effective.

A *balanced meal* is one which provides adequate amounts of protein and of all the minerals and vitamins as well as energy. It should also provide dietary fibre, and should be limited in its fat, sugar and salt contents – particularly if these are likely to be amply supplied from other sources during the day. At least one balanced meal should be eaten every day.

The main sources of each nutrient are discussed in Chapters 2, 3, 4, 7 and 8, the detailed composition of a range of foods is given in Appendix 2. Most foods contain a wide variety of nutrients, and most minerals and vitamins are present in a wide variety of common foods. Thus the simplest way to meet nutritional standards is to eat a varied diet containing a wide selection of different types of food.

Experience and custom have influenced food choice in such a way that traditional meals are generally nutritionally satisfactory as well as good to eat; nevertheless to be sure that this is maintained, now that we rely to a greater extent on snacks and convenience foods, certain general rules can be followed:

(a) Each meal should contain some foods rich in *protein*, such as meat, poultry, fish, cheese, eggs, milk, bread or other cereal product, nuts, peas or beans.

(b) Each main meal should contain plenty of *fruit* and *vegetables*, which are good sources of some vitamins and minerals not commonly found in other foods.

(c) Foods rich in energy should be eaten only in amounts which will satisfy appetite and maintain correct body weight. Such foods include butter and margarine (which also provide vitamins A and D), bread and other cereals (which also provide protein, minerals, vitamins and dietary fibre) and only then jam, cakes, biscuits and other foods rich in sugar and fat.

The total daily intake of each of the major nutrients which is recommended for groups of people of different ages and occupations is given on page 56, and these figures may be used as targets when planning diets. The total amount of fat should not provide more than 35 per cent of the energy in the diet, nor saturated plus *trans* fatty acids more than 15 per cent of the energy except for small children (N.B. human breast milk derives 54 per cent of its energy from fat and 26 per cent from saturated fatty acids). By implication, the total carbohydrate in the diet should provide about 55 per cent of the dietary energy, but there are as yet no comparable recommendations for the proportions of sugars or dietary fibre nor for the amount of sodium to be eaten by people of each sex at different ages. In practice it will be found that certain meals such as traditional Sunday lunch are likely to be rich in many nutrients whereas others, including breakfasts for many people, will prove a counterbalance. It is the *total* nutrient intake over at least one day (as in the example on page 100), and preferably a week, that should be assessed; and even then it is the adequacy of the diet in the longer term which is really important for health.

Planning meals in relation to cost

Within this general framework it is usually necessary to consider the relative cost of different sources of nutrients. Allowance must also be made for the effects of cooking on nutritive value (see page 66).

Great savings in the cost of eating can be made with a thorough knowledge of food composition and nutritional value for money. For example, cheaper cuts of meat have practically the same nutritional value as the more expensive cuts although they may take longer to cook. Many meat products also provide good nutritional value for money. Again, cheaper fatty fish such as mackerel has a similar nutritional value to an expensive fatty fish such as salmon. The cheaper fresh vegetables such as cabbage, carrots and potatoes are often much better value for money than many canned or frozen vegetables. Fresh citrus fruits are very convenient sources of vitamin C and are also fairly cheap. Cheese and eggs can take the place of meat in a main course.

Section 3 of Appendix 3 (page 117) shows how the amounts of protein, vitamins or any nutrients bought for one penny can be calculated for any food by using the food composition tables and the price of the food. The precise relationship between foods will vary according to the time of year and current prices, but Table 31 gives a general idea of some *cheap* sources of certain nutrients. It is important to realise that a cheap source of one nutrient may not be a cheap food in the context of the whole diet, as with sugar where only one nutrient is supplied. Bread, pasta, rice, breakfast cereals, milk, cheese, offals, potatoes, peas and beans, on the other hand, all supply several nutrients cheaply and are thus very good value for money.

Planning meals for the week ahead is most important in food budgeting. Careful shopping, correct preparation and storage of food, and a good standard of cookery all play a part in using the available money to the best advantage.

Table 31. **Cheap sources of energy and nutrients (in approximate[1] order, with the cheapest first)**

Energy	Lard, margarine, vegetable oil, sugar, white bread, butter, brown or wholemeal bread, old potatoes, pasta, rice, biscuits, breakfast cereals.
Protein	White bread, brown or wholemeal bread, pasta, liver, eggs, baked beans, cheese, milk, chicken, rice, frozen peas, old potatoes.
Carbohydrate	Sugar, white bread, old potatoes, rice, pasta, brown or wholemeal bread, breakfast cereals, new potatoes, biscuits, baked beans, ice cream.
Calcium	Milk, cheese, white bread, brown bread, wholemeal bread, carrots, ice cream, biscuits.
Iron	Liver, fortified breakfast cereals, brown or wholemeal bread, white bread, baked beans, new potatoes, old potatoes, eggs, biscuits.
Vitamin A	Liver, carrots, margarine, butter, eggs, milk, cheese.
Thiamin	Fortified breakfast cereals, old potatoes, new potatoes, brown or wholemeal bread, white bread, frozen peas, pork, liver, bacon and ham.
Riboflavin	Liver, fortified breakfast cereals, milk, cheese, brown or wholemeal bread, old potatoes.
Niacin	Liver, breakfast cereals, white bread, old potatoes, new potatoes, chicken, sausages, frozen peas.
Vitamin C	Fruit juices, oranges, old potatoes, new potatoes, tomatoes, fresh green vegetables, frozen peas.
Vitamin D	Margarine, fatty fish, eggs, fortified breakfast cereals, liver, butter.
Dietary fibre	Dried beans, All bran, wholemeal bread, baked beans, white bread, potatoes, whole grain breakfast cereals and pasta.

[1] When harvests are badly affected by weather conditions, the nutritional value for money provided by some of these foods may decline.

13 Needs of particular groups of people

Infants and young children

Infants are unique in that they must rely on a single food, milk, to satisfy all their nutritional needs. Breast milk is ideal for several reasons:
  (a) All the nutrients are present in the right amount for human infants, and in a readily absorbed form. Those nutrients which are low, such as iron and copper, are those which are already stored in large amounts in the infant's liver.
  (b) It contains several natural agents which protect against disease.
  (c) It is clean, cannot be prepared incorrectly, and does not cause allergies.

A mother should therefore try to breast feed her baby for at least 2 weeks, and ideally for 4-6 months. Few mothers are unable to breast feed. Some cannot for medical reasons and some prefer not to do so; then formulas, usually based on cows' milk, which has been modified so that it is more like human milk, can be used. Because the immature kidneys of young infants are unable to adapt to high concentrations of protein and some minerals it is very important to make up these feeds exactly according to the instructions so that they are not overconcentrated. In hot weather extra water may be needed but sugary drinks and juices can harm the developing teeth.

Solid foods should not be introduced before 4 months of age. There is no advantage to the baby to do so and there may be some risks of developing allergies and of becoming obese. From about 6 months onwards the mother may gradually introduce infant cereal foods, pureed fruit and vegetables, egg yolk, and even finely divided meat (using no added salt or sugar). By about 12-18 months, the infant can eat a mixed diet not very different from that of the rest of the family. Milk will continue to be very important but less will be drunk as more solid foods are eaten.

Drops containing vitamins A, C and D may also be useful as may fluoride supplements in areas where the drinking water is low in fluoride.

Schoolchildren

Schoolchildren are growing fast and are also very active. Table 24 on page 56 gives the recommended intakes of energy and nutrients for groups of children of different ages and shows that these are high in relation to their body size compared with those of adults. For example, the recommendations for 7-8 year old girls for energy, protein and thiamin are nearly as high as those for grown women in most occupations, and for calcium is even higher. The big appetites of some children usually reflect a real nutritional need rather than greed. Because of their smaller size compared with adults, and correspondingly small stomachs, it is important that children should eat meals which are not too bulky. Bread, milk, cheese, meat, fish, liver, eggs, fruit and green vegetables and potatoes are excellent sources of a number of nutrients. Milk, whether whole, semi-skimmed or skimmed, is one of the best sources of calcium, riboflavin and protein. Children should be taught sensible eating habits from an early age: biscuits, sweets, soft drinks, chips and crisps should not be allowed to displace other more useful foods too often, either at home or at school.

Adolescents

The nutrient needs of adolescents are higher in many respects than those of any other group. Healthy adolescents have very big appetites and it is important that they should satisfy them with food of high nutritional value in the form of well balanced meals (page 90) rather than by too many snacks rich in fat, sugar or salt. Obesity among schoolchildren is common and this may continue into adult life. It is more sensible to prevent obesity than try to correct it by periodically eating little or no food: excessive dieting can be dangerous (page 23). There is also evidence that adolescent obesity is partly due to a general decrease in physical activity and hence in energy expenditure rather than to an excessive energy intake. A knowledge of nutrition and the incentive to apply this knowledge in practice is likely to benefit the health of young people for the rest of their lives. Dental decay is very common in British schoolchildren; sweet and sticky foods and snacks eaten between meals are one cause of this (page 9).

Adolescent girls who become pregnant are at particular risk, needing additional nutrients for their baby's growth as well as for their own.

Adults

Many adults in Britain are more likely to be at risk of overnutrition than of undernutrition. Those adults who wish to reduce their intakes of energy or of fat and saturated fatty acids to reduce their risk of a premature heart attack will find information throughout this Manual which will help them to achieve this. Middle-aged men are at particular risk, but any diet will be easier to follow if it is shared with other members of the family or with friends. There is also information for those who wish to reduce their intakes of sugars and salt and to increase their intake of dietary fibre.

In general, such diets are similar to long-term slimming diets (page 96), except that extra cereal products including bread, rice and pasta, and potatoes, will be needed to make good the energy lost from the reduction in fats and sugars. These foods will also contribute dietary fibre, but may add

94

to the total salt intake unless less salt is used on the plate and in the preparation of vegetables and meat dishes. It is always wise to evaluate the whole diet before making any changes, so that the intake of other nutrients as well as the nutrient of concern, and the main foods which contribute to these intakes, are known. There would be little point, for example, in reducing an individual's fat intake further if his diet is already low in fat; or of reducing his intake of a favourite food if it contributes little to his overall fat intake; or of reducing fat intakes if the foods eaten instead are rich in sugars or salt.

It is also important to keep alcohol intake under control.

Pregnancy and Lactation

A woman's nutritional needs increase during pregnancy and lactation (page 56). This is not only because her diet must provide for the growth and development of her child (as below), but also because other physiological changes occur to ensure that sufficient nutrients are available for the child such as the laying down of new tissues in the woman's own body. Much of the weight gain durng the early part of pregnancy is due to the accumulation of fat which provides an energy store to meet the additional demands of the growing fetus and the breast-fed infant.

Approximate weight of an infant at various ages

Conception	0 kg
4½ months pregnancy	0.5 kg
9 months pregnancy (birth)	3.5 kg
4½ months after birth	7 kg

It is most important that the mother's diet contains sufficient energy, protein, iron, calcium, folic acid and vitamins C and D (and liquid during lactation) for building the baby's muscular tissues, bones and teeth, and for the formation of haemoglobin; if it does not, her own stores of nutrients may be reduced. Some good sources of these nutrients are given in Part 1. In practice most of these extra nutrients will be obtained simply by satisfying the appetite with a good mixed diet including plenty of milk, cheese, liver, bread, fruit and vegetables, but special supplements of iron and folic acid are often recommended during pregnancy and tablets containing calcium, iodine and vitamins A, C and D are also available to those in need. A good knowledge of nutrition is invaluable at this stage and will also help the mother to teach sound eating habits to her child in due course.

Old people

There is very little difference between the nutritional requirements of the elderly and the younger adult (page 56), but because the elderly tend to be less active after the age of 75, their average energy requirements are less. The recommendations for energy and for those nutrients needed for its utilization are therefore reduced, and for some, dietary adjustments such as a reduction in fat consumption will be necessary to avoid an increase in weight. Those with poor teeth, arthritis or other physical disabilities or poor appetites who live alone should be encouraged to cook at least one meal a day of good nutritional quality, and to supplement this with foods such as milk, breakfast cereals, eggs, cheese, bread, and fruits rich in vitamin C, which need little preparation. For the housebound who do not have the benefit of sunlight a good dietary source of vitamin D such as margarine, eggs or fatty fish (e.g., sardines, kippers) is important. Foods rich in dietary fibre may also help to prevent constipation.

Slimmers

Energy needs and food consumption have been discussed in Chapter 5.

Planning a slimming diet is a matter of individual preference. Essentially, the energy intake should be cut down by up to 1,000 kilocalories (4 MJ) each day while other nutrients should still reach recommended levels. It is often convenient to cut out fatty and sugary foods such as sweets, preserves, biscuits and puddings as well as alcohol as these tend to be sources of energy rather than nutrients. Fat can be trimmed from meat, and foods can be boiled or grilled and not fried. Foods high in water or dietary fibre can induce feelings of fullness and so help to reduce the desire for more food.

Effective slimming diets are all basically low energy or 'low calorie' diets, though they vary in how this is achieved. A good plan is to base meals on a modest helping of lean meat, fish, eggs or cheese with liberal amounts of fruits and vegetables and small amounts of bread and potatoes. Eating three or four meals a day gives better results than eating the same amount of food at one or two meals only; breakfast should be included. As it may take several months to reach the desired weight, a slimming diet should be sensible and palatable enough to be tolerated for this length of time. After this, a diet of reduced energy content may still be needed to maintain the correct weight. Cranky diets based on one or two foods only or on powdered protein with added minerals and vitamins may be successful in the short term but are hard to adhere to as they are unrealistic, dull, and sometimes expensive; they can also be nutritionally dangerous.

It can be very difficult to reduce food intake. Some people turn to food for comfort and others must attend social functions where dieting is difficult. The wide range of reduced fat and reduced energy foods now available may be helpful. Keeping to a diet can sometimes be made easier by joining a slimmers' group.

Vegetarians

Vegetarians do not eat meat and most do not eat fish, but the majority consume some animal products – the most important of which are milk, cheese and eggs. Such diets may be rather bulky and lower in energy than a mixed diet because most vegetables have a high water content but, in general, their nutritional values are very similar to those of mixed diets.

A much smaller group, *vegans*, eat no foods of animal origin at all. Man's nutrient requirements with the exception of vitamin B_{12} (page 48) can be met by a diet composed entirely of plant foods but to do so it must be carefully planned using a wide selection of foods. A mixture of plant proteins derived from cereals, peas, beans and nuts will provide sufficient protein of good quality, but special care is needed to ensure that sufficient energy, calcium, iron, riboflavin, vitamin B_{12} and vitamin D are also available. Yeast extract is a good source of some of the B-vitamins including vitamin B_{12} which are otherwise found mainly in animal foods.

Organic and Health Foods

All foods, being derived from plants or animals, are organic; and all foods, because they provide nutrients, are conducive to health when eaten as part of a balanced diet as described in this Manual. The words have, however, come to acquire the restricted meaning of foods grown without the use of inorganic fertilizers, pesticides or herbicides, and either not processed or processed without the use of additives. These substances must be used if enough food for our dense urban population is to be grown and distributed economically, and their use is controlled by legislation (page 121). Furthermore, they have little effect on nutritional value, which is largely determined by the species of plant or animal.

People who choose to restrict their diet in this way, should, like vegetarians or anyone else whose diet is limited, take extra care to ensure that they obtain enough of all the nutrients. Shops which sell such food often sell vitamin and mineral supplements too, presumably for this reason. In extreme cases, such as zen macrobiotic diets where little but whole grain cereals are eaten, intakes of calcium, iron, vitamin B_{12} and vitamin C are likely to be too low for health.

Immigrants

Immigrant communities in Britain which retain their traditional diets and customs (see Table 32) may have special dietary problems. In particular, Asian groups may have very low intakes of vitamin D. Because exposure to sunlight (especially by women and children) may also be low due to customs of dress and because they tend to remain indoors, rickets and osteomalacia sometimes develop. Good sources of vitamin D (page 52) should therefore

Table 32. Dietary restrictions practised by religious and ethnic groups

HINDUS	No beef	Mostly vegetarian; fish rarely eaten; no alcohol	Periods of fasting common.
MUSLIMS	No pork	Meat must be 'Halal'; no shellfish eaten; no alcohol	Regular fasting, including Ramadan for 1 month.
SIKHS	No beef	Meat must be killed by 'one blow to the head'; no alcohol	Generally less rigid eating restrictions than Hindus and Muslims.
JEWS	No pork	Meat must be kosher; only fish with scales and fins eaten	Meat and dairy foods must not be consumed together.
RASTAFARIANS	No animal products, except milk may be consumed	Foods must be 'I-tal' or alive, so no canned or processed foods eaten; no salt added; no coffee or alcohol	Food should be 'organic'.

Halal meat must be bled to death and dedicated to God by a Muslim present at the killing. Kosher meat must be bled to death in the presence of a Rabbi and then be soaked and salted.

Orthodox members may adhere to all the restrictions of their religion or ethnic group. Others may adhere to only the major restrictions, especially where they are an immigrant in a foreign country.

be included in sufficient quantity in the diet and vitamin supplements may be necessary. The iron content of some traditional diets is also low.

Diabetics

Diabetes is a metabolic disorder which reduces the ability of the body to control the amount of glucose in the blood (page 32). It is important for diabetics to avoid the rapid rises in blood glucose which result from eating large amounts of readily absorbed carbohydrate, but this requires control rather than a reduction in total carbohydrate intake. Indeed, many Asian diabetics live well with 60 per cent or more of their diet as carbohydrate from rice or chapatis, and traditional low carbohydrate diets, being high in fat, may have contributed to the prevalence of heart disease in British diabetics. It is most important for diabetics to control their weight since obesity reduces the body's ability to metabolize glucose. Otherwise they should eat diets similar to those recommended for any other adult.

Other special diets

The principles set out in this Manual hold in general for all healthy individuals. There are, however, a few people who possess personal idiosyncrasies causing reactions to certain foods, for example, eggs, shellfish or strawberries. In conditions such as coeliac disease (page 17) or lactose intolerance (page 9), a special diet should be followed, and, when certain drugs are taken, the avoidance of some foods such as cheese is necessary. These allergies and illnesses are a medical rather than a nutritional problem.

Summary: assessing the adequacy of a diet

It is important not only that all the essential nutrients should be present in the foods eaten, but also that they should be present in the amounts required by different people. To find out whether a particular diet is nutritionally adequate, three things must be known:
(a) What foods were eaten?
(b) How much of each food was eaten?
(c) What kind of person or people ate the foods? Were they men, women, adolescents or children, and were they very active or sedentary? Were any of the women pregnant or nursing a baby?

When the answers to these questions are known, daily nutrient intakes can then be compared with the amounts recommended for health (page 56) and any other appropriate guidelines. It must however be emphasized that the mineral and vitamin recommendations are high enough to cover the needs of practically all healthy people; therefore it is only when an individual is consistently obtaining less than this recommended intake that there could be any cause for concern.

Three important methods of measuring food consumption are:
(a) Measuring the amount of food purchased by, for example, a family during one week. When the amount of food bought is recorded, it is important to follow up by finding out how much of it is eaten, how much goes into or out of the store cupboard or freezer, how many people ate it, and how much is wasted in preparing meals and on the plate (page 89).
(b) Recalling, preferably with expert help, all the foods eaten in the previous 24 hours or 3 days. This is the least time-consuming method, but it is easy to forget important foods and hard to estimate quantities accurately.
(c) Weighing all the foods eaten or drunk over a long enough period (usually a whole week). Provided that the diet is not changed to accommodate the complex recording procedure, this should be the most precise method of assessing the value of anyone's diet.

It is easy to determine the weights of standard or pre-packaged items, and for meals served in canteens or restaurants it may be possible to weigh all the components of duplicates of the meal. More care is needed to evaluate variable domestic items such as stews. It is also important to remember that the nutrient content of foods may vary from the average values shown in this Manual.

As an example of the way in which a diet can be evaluated, the daily pattern of snacks and meals which might have been eaten by a young man in a sedentary occupation has been set out in a systematic way in Table 33.

Table 33. **Menu for one day for a young sedentary man**

Breakfast	wt (g)	Evening meal	wt (g)
Orange juice	112	Beef sausages	120
2 fried eggs	110	Chips	100
White bread	30	Frozen peas	80
Butter	7	1 apple	120
Marmalade	10		
1 cup of tea			
Milk with tea	28		
Sugar with tea	10	Snacks throughout the day	wt (g)
		1 cup of tea	
Lunch (sandwiches)	wt (g)	Milk with tea	28
		Sugar with tea	10
White bread	120	Chocolate	50
Margarine	28	2 digestive biscuits	28
Ham	50	1 pt beer	570
1 can carbonated drink	330		

The nutrients provided by these quantities of each of these foods must be calculated using food tables such as that in Appendix 2. The results can be summarized meal by meal as in Table 34, or the contribution of each food to each nutrient can be listed if the evaluation covers only a short period.

The intakes of each nutrient can then be compared with the amounts recommended for such a person, and with an understanding of the principles set out in this Manual the significance of any departures from these recommendations can then be assessed. In this instance:

(a) The *energy* intake is very close to that recommended for a man of his age and occupational activity. However, many sedentary men now eat less, and it is possible that he may gain weight if such a meal pattern were eaten regularly.

(b) The proportion of the total energy intake derived from *protein* was 10.9 per cent, which is acceptable, and that from *fat* was 40.6 per cent. As the recommended fat intake refers only to *food* (i.e. excluding the energy from alcoholic drinks), this intake has been recalculated as 43.4 per cent of the food energy. This should be reduced to 35 per cent by eating lower fat meals on other days; alternatively, since much of this man's fat intake was derived from fried foods and from

Table 34. **Nutrient content of a menu for a young sedentary man** (see Table 33)

	Energy kcal	Protein g	Fat g	Carbo-hydrate g	Dietary fibre[1] g	Calcium mg	Iron mg	Sodium mg	Thiamin mg	Vitamin C mg
Breakfast	502	19.6	28.8	43.9	1.3	149.4	3.7	479	0.24	39.6
Lunch	689	18.1	30.3	91.3	4.9	142.3	2.6	1,583	0.52	0
Evening meal	656	24.2	32.2	72.0	15.1	127.4	4.3	1,359	0.48	24.4
Snacks	665	6.9	22.1	73.9	1.4	210.4	1.7	276	0.10	0.4
TOTAL	2,512	68.9	113.3	281.0	22.7	629.5	12.4	3,696	1.35	64.4
Recommended intake (DHSS 1979)	2,510	63	—	—	—	500	10		1.0	30

[1] Dietary fibre values will be lower if a different analytical method is used (page 8).

101

confectionery items, it would be reduced if the eggs and potatoes had been boiled. The advice for those people with high fat intakes who derive most of that fat from meats, milk, cheese or snacks would, of course, be different.

(c) The intake of *dietary fibre* would be increased if more fruit and vegetables were eaten or if the sandwiches had been made from wholemeal bread.

(d) *Mineral* and *vitamin* intakes were well above those recommended by the Department of Health and Social Security. In general it is easier for men to achieve this than it is for women: men usually eat more food and thus obtain more minerals, vitamins and dietary fibre (but also more of the filling fats and carbohydrates). The sodium intake was, however, high and it would be inadvisable for this man to add further salt to any of his meals at the table.

APPENDICES

1 Common measures and conversion factors

Although the labels of most pre-packed foods give their weight in grams, many fresh foods are weighed in Imperial units and many individuals still use pounds weight, pints, inches, etc. Furthermore energy has long been measured in *calories*, but the SI units *joules* are also being used. The conversion factors below show the relationships between these units.

WEIGHT

1 milligram (mg)	= 1,000 micrograms (μg)	
1 gram (g)	= 1,000 mg	= 0.035 ounces (oz)
1 kilogram (kg)	= 1,000 g	= 2.20 pounds (lb)
1 oz	= 28.35 g	
1 lb	= 453.6 g	

VOLUME

1 litre	= 1,000 millilitres (ml)	= 1.76 pints (pt)
1 pt	= 20 fluid oz	= 568 ml

LENGTH

1 metre (m)	= 100 centimetres (cm)	= 1,000 millimetres (mm)
		= 39.4 inches (in)
1 in	= 2.54 cm	
1 foot (ft)	= 0.3048 m	

ENERGY

1 kilojoule (kJ)	= 1,000 joules (J)	
1 megajoule (MJ)	= 1,000 kJ	= 239 kilocalories (kcal)
1 kcal	= 4.184 kJ	

2 Composition of food

Typical values for the amounts of a number of nutrients in a wide variety of raw and cooked foods are shown in the following table. Each value is the amount per 100 grams of the edible part of the food as described.

The information is based partly on the 4th revised edition of McCance and Widdowson's *The Composition of Foods* (1978), which gives details of more foods and more nutrients than are shown here, and partly on more recent analyses done for the Ministry of Agriculture, Fisheries and Food. Individual samples of food can differ considerably depending on the season of the year, the recipe, cooking method, and many other factors. For pre-packaged foods, therefore, any information given on the label by the manufacturers should be more appropriate for that particular product than the more general values in this Appendix.

Allowance may need to be made for wastage in foods that are weighed raw. The values given here predict the proportion of each food *as listed* that cannot be eaten. Thus for raw lamb it is the amount of bone likely to be in a cut or joint to be cooked, but for slices of roast lamb there would be no wastage. Some individuals may, however, choose not to eat some of the fat or to discard any parts of a fruit that are bruised, and an additional allowance may have to be made for this.

The energy value of each food is given in kilojoules (kJ) as well as in kilocalories (kcal), and both have been calculated from the protein, fat and carbohydrate content as on page 24. Two of the vitamins are given in the form of equivalents; these are vitamin A, as retinol equivalents (page 42), and niacin, which includes the contribution from tryptophan (page 47). They are thus expressed in the same form as in the *Recommended Daily Amounts of Food Energy and Nutrients for Groups of People in the United Kingdom* (page 56). Available carbohydrate is given as its monosaccharide equivalent (page 6). Appendix 3 provides examples of the use of this Table.

Table 1. **Composition per 100 g (raw edible weight except where stated)**

No.	Food	Inedible waste	Energy		Protein	Fat	Carbo-hydrate (as mono saccharide
		%	kcal	kJ	g	g	g
	Milk						
1	Cream – double	0	447	1,841	1.5	48.2	2.0
2	Cream – single	0	195	806	2.4	19.3	3.2
3	Milk, liquid, whole	0	65	272	3.2	3.9	4.6
4	Milk, liquid, skimmed	0	32	137	3.4	0.1	4.7
5	Milk, condensed whole, sweetened	0	170	709	8.5	10.2	11.7
6	Milk, whole, evaporated	0	149	620	8.4	9.4	8.1
7	Milk, dried, skimmed	0	339	1,442	36.1	0.6	50.4
8	Yogurt, low fat, natural	0	65	276	5.1	0.8	10.0
9	Yogurt, low fat, fruit	0	89	382	4.1	0.7	17.9
	Cheese						
10	Cheddar	0	406	1,682	26.0	33.5	0
11	Cottage	0	96	402	13.6	4.0	1.4
12	Cheese spread	0	283	1,173	18.3	22.9	0.9
13	Feta	0	245	1,017	16.5	19.9	0
14	Brie	0	300	1,246	22.8	23.2	0
	Meat						
15	Bacon, rashers, raw	11	339	1,402	13.9	31.5	0
16	Bacon, rashers, grilled	0	393	1,632	28.1	31.2	0
17	Beef, average, raw	17	313	1,296	16.6	27.4	0
18	Beef, mince, stewed	0	229	955	23.1	15.2	0
19	Beef, stewing steak, raw	4	176	736	20.2	10.6	0
20	Beef, stewing steak, cooked	0	223	932	30.9	11.0	0
21	Black pudding, fried	0	305	1,270	12.9	21.9	15.0
22	Chicken, raw	41	194	809	19.7	12.8	0
23	Chicken, roast, meat and skin	0	213	888	24.4	12.8	0
24	Chicken, roast, meat only	0	148	621	24.8	5.4	0
25	Corned beef	0	202	844	25.9	10.9	0
26	Ham	0	166	690	16.4	11.1	0
27	Kidney, pigs, raw	6	86	363	15.5	2.7	0
28	Kidney, pigs, fried	0	202	848	29.2	9.5	0
29	Lamb, average, raw	23	295	1,223	16.2	25.6	0
30	Lamb, roast	0	266	1,106	26.1	17.9	0
31	Liver, lambs, raw	0	140	587	20.3	6.2	0.8
32	Liver, lambs, fried	0	237	989	30.1	12.9	0
33	Luncheon meat	0	266	1,153	12.9	23.8	3.3
34	Paté, average	0	347	1,436	13.7	31.9	1.4
35	Pork, average, raw	26	297	1,231	16.9	25.5	0
36	Pork chop, cooked	26	332	1,380	28.5	24.2	0
37	Sausage, beef, cooked	0	267	1,114	12.9	17.7	15.0
38	Sausage, pork, cooked	0	317	1,318	13.6	24.5	11.2
39	Steak & kidney pie	0	274	1,146	9.3	17.1	22.2
40	Turkey, roast, meat & skin	0	189	793	26.2	9.4	0

ater	Calcium mg	Iron mg	Sodium mg	Vitamin A (retinol equivalent) µg	Thiamin mg	Riboflavin mg	Niacin equivalent mg	Vitamin C mg	No.
9	50	0.2	30	500	0.02	0.08	0.4	1	1
2	79	0.3	40	155	0.03	0.12	0.8	1	2
8	103	0.1	50	56	0.05	0.17	0.9	1.5	3
1	108	0.1	50	1	0.05	0.18	0.9	1.5	4
0	270	0.2	140	123	0.09	0.46	2.3	4.1	5
9	260	0.3	170	125	0.07	0.42	2.1	1.5	6
3	1,230	0.3	510	550	0.38	0.16	9.5	13.2	7
6	200	0.1	80	12	0.06	0.25	1.2	0.8	8
7	150	0.1	70	12	0.05	0.21	1.2	0.7	9
7	800	0.4	610	363	0.04	0.50	6.2	0	10
9	60	0.1	450	41	0.02	0.19	3.3	0	11
1	510	0.7	1,170	198	0.02	0.24	0.1	0	12
6	384	0.2	1,260	270	0.03	0.11	4.2	0	13
8	380	0.8	1,410	238	0.09	0.60	6.2	0	14
1	7	0.6	1,340	0	0.45	0.14	6.5	0	15
4	14	1.3	2,404	0	0.57	0.27	12.5	0	16
5	7	1.9	70	10	0.05	0.23	6.9	0	17
9	18	3.1	320	0	0.05	0.33	9.3	0	18
9	8	2.1	72	0	0.06	0.23	8.5	0	19
7	15	3.0	360	0	0.03	0.33	10.2	0	20
4	35	20.0	1,210	0	0.09	0.07	3.8	0	21
7	9	0.7	75	0	0.11	0.13	9.6	0	22
2	13	0.5	90	0	0.05	0.19	13.6	0	23
8	9	0.8	81	0	0.08	0.19	12.8	0	24
9	27	2.4	854	0	0	0.20	9.1	0	25
7	4	0.6	1,405	0	0.54	0.20	6.3	0	26
0	10	6.4	200	160	0.56	2.58	11.1	6.5	27
8	12	9.1	220	220	0.41	3.70	20.1	11.9	28
6	7	1.4	71	0	0.09	0.21	7.1	0	29
5	8	2.5	65	0	0.12	0.31	11.0	0	30
0	6	7.5	73	19,900	0.39	4.64	20.7	19.2	31
4	8	10.9	83	30,500	0.38	5.65	24.7	18.6	32
4	39	1.0	913	0	0.06	0.15	3.9	0	33
7	14	8.2	762	8,300	0.14	1.32	4.3	0	34
7	8	0.9	65	0	0.49	0.20	8.9	0	35
6	11	1.2	84	0	0.66	0.20	11.0	0	36
8	68	1.6	1,095	0	0	0.14	9.0	0	37
5	54	1.5	1,075	0	0.01	0.16	7.2	0	38
4	47	1.8	402	0	0.12	0.25	4.9	0	39
3	7	0.9	70	0	0.09	0.16	12.2	0	40

Composition per 100 g

No.	Food	Inedible waste	Energy		Protein	Fat	Carbo-hydrate (as mono sacchari
		%	kcal	kJ	g	g	g
	Fish						
41	White fish, filleted	3	77	324	17.1	0.9	0
42	Cod, fried	0	235	982	19.6	14.3	7.5
43	Fish fingers, raw	0	178	749	12.6	7.5	16.1
44	Herrings, whole	46	251	1,040	16.8	20.4	0
45	Mackerel	40	282	1,170	19.0	22.9	0
46	Pilchards, canned in tomato sauce	0	126	531	18.8	5.4	0.7
47	Sardines, canned in oil, fish only	0	217	906	23.7	18.6	0
48	Tuna in oil	0	289	1,202	22.8	22.0	0
49	Prawns, boiled	0	107	451	22.6	1.8	0
	Eggs						
50	Eggs, boiled	12	147	612	12.3	10.9	0
51	Eggs, fried	0	232	961	14.1	19.5	0
	Fats						
52	Butter	0	740	3,041	0.4	82.0	0
53	Lard, cooking fat, dripping	0	892	3,667	0	99.1	0
54	Low fat spread	0	366	1,506	0	40.7	0
55	Margarine, average	0	730	3,000	0.1	81.0	0
56	Cooking and salad oil	0	899	3,696	0	99.9	0
	Preserves, etc.						
57	Chocolate, milk	0	529	2,214	8.4	30.3	59.4
58	Honey	0	288	1,229	0.4	0	76.4
59	Jam	0	262	1,116	0.5	0	69.2
60	Marmalade	0	261	1,114	0.1	0	69.5
61	Sugar, white	0	394	1,680	0	0	105.3
62	Syrup	0	298	1,269	0.3	0	79.0
63	Peppermints	0	392	1,670	0.5	0.7	102.2
	Vegetables						
64	Aubergines	23	14	62	0.7	0	3.1
65	Baked beans	0	81	345	4.8	0.6	15.1
66	Beans, runner, boiled	1	19	83	1.9	0.2	2.7
67	Beans, red kidney, raw	0	272	1,159	22.1	1.7	45.0
68	Beans, soya, boiled	0	141	592	12.4	6.4	9.0
69	Beetroot, boiled	0	44	189	1.8	0	9.9
70	Brussels sprouts, boiled	0	18	75	2.8	0	1.7
71	Cabbage, raw	43	22	92	2.8	0	2.8
72	Cabbage, boiled	0	15	66	1.7	0	2.3
73	Carrots, old	4	23	98	0.7	0	5.4
74	Cauliflower, cooked	0	9	40	1.6	0	0.8
75	Celery	27	8	36	0.9	0	1.3
76	Courgettes, raw	13	29	122	1.6	0.4	5.0

ter	Calcium	Iron	Sodium	Vitamin A (retinol equivalent)	Thiamin	Riboflavin	Niacin equivalent	Vitamin C	No.
	mg	mg	mg	μg	mg	mg	mg	mg	
2	22	0.5	99	1	0.07	0.09	6.0	0	41
7	80	0.5	100	0	0.06	0.07	4.9	0	42
4	43	0.7	320	0.2	0.09	0.06	3.5	0	43
4	33	0.8	67	46	0	0.18	7.2	0	44
7	24	1.0	130	45	0.09	0.35	11.6	0	45
4	300	2.7	370	8	0.02	0.29	11.1	0	46
8	550	2.9	650	7	0.04	0.36	12.6	0	47
5	7	1.1	420	0	0.04	0.11	17.2	0	48
0	150	1.1	1,590	0	0.03	0.03	7.4	0	49
5	52	2.0	140	190	0.09	0.47	3.7	0	50
3	64	2.5	220	140	0.07	0.42	4.2	0	51
5	15	0.2	870	985	0	0	0.1	0	52
1	1	0.1	2	0	0	0	0	0	53
4	0	0	690	900	0	0	0	0	54
6	4	0.3	800	860	0	0	0.1	0	55
0	0	0	0	0	0	0	0	0	56
2	220	1.6	120	6.6	0.10	0.23	1.6	0	57
3	5	0.4	11	0	0	0.05	0.2	0	58
0	18	1.2	14	2	0	0	0	10	59
8	35	0.6	18	8	0	0	0	10	60
0	2	0	0	0	0	0	0	0	61
8	26	1.5	270	0	0	0	0	0	62
0	7	0.2	9	0	0	0	0	0	63
3	10	0.4	3	0	0.05	0.03	1.0	5	64
4	48	1.4	550	12	0.08	0.06	1.3	0	65
1	22	0.7	1	67	0.03	0.07	0.8	5	66
1	140	6.7	40	0	0.54	0.18	5.5	0	67
7	145	2.5	15	0	0.26	0.16	3.4	0	68
3	30	0.4	64	0	0.02	0.04	0.4	5	69
2	25	0.5	2	67	0.06	0.10	0.9	40	70
3	57	0.6	7	50	0.06	0.05	0.8	55	71
3	38	0.4	4	50	0.03	0.03	0.5	20	72
0	48	0.6	95	2,000	0.06	0.05	0.7	6	73
5	18	0.4	4	5	0.06	0.06	0.8	20	74
4	52	0.6	140	0	0.03	0.03	0.5	7	75
2	30	1.5	1	58	0.05	0.09	0.6	16	76

Composition per 100 g

No.	Food	Inedible waste %	Energy kcal	kJ	Protein g	Fat g	Carbo-hydrate (as mono saccharide) g
77	Cucumber	23	10	43	0.6	0.1	1.8
78	Lentils, cooked	0	99	420	7.6	0.5	17.0
79	Lettuce	30	12	51	1.0	0.4	1.2
80	Mushrooms	25	13	53	1.8	0.6	0
81	Onion	3	23	99	0.9	0	5.2
82	Parsnips, cooked	0	56	238	1.3	0	13.5
83	Peas, frozen, boiled	0	72	307	6.0	0.9	10.7
84	Peas, canned processed	0	86	366	6.9	0.7	18.9
85	Peppers, green	14	12	51	0.9	0	2.2
86	Potatoes	10[1] 20[2]	74	315	2.0	0.2	17.1
87	Potatoes, boiled	0	76	322	1.8	0.1	18.0
88	Potato crisps	0	533	2,224	6.3	35.9	49.3
89	Potatoes, fried (chips)	0	234	983	3.6	10.2	34.0
90	Potatoes, oven chips	0	162	687	3.2	4.2	29.8
91	Potatoes, roast	0	150	632	3.0	4.5	25.9
92	Spinach, boiled	0	30	128	5.1	0.5	1.4
93	Sweetcorn, canned	0	85	379	2.9	1.2	16.8
94	Sweet potato	14	91	387	1.2	0.6	21.5
95	Tomatoes, fresh	0	14	60	0.9	0	2.8
96	Turnips, cooked	0	14	60	0.7	0.3	2.3
97	Watercress	23	14	61	2.9	0	0.7
98	Yam, boiled	0	119	508	1.6	0.1	29.8
	Fruit						
99	Apples	20	46	196	0.3	0	11.9
100	Apricots, canned in syrup	0	106	452	0.5	0	27.7
101	Apricots, dried	0	182	772	4.8	0	43.4
102	Avocado pear	29	223	922	4.2	22.2	1.8
103	Bananas	40	76	326	1.1	0	19.2
104	Blackcurrants	2	28	121	0.9	0	6.6
105	Cherries	13	47	201	0.6	0	11.9
106	Dates, dried	14	248	1,056	2.0	0	63.9
107	Figs, dried	0	213	908	3.6	0	52.9
108	Gooseberries, cooked, unsweetened	0	14	62	0.9	0	2.9
109	Grapes	5	63	268	0.6	0	16.1
110	Grapefruit	50	22	95	0.6	0	5.3
111	Lemon juice	64	7	31	0.3	0	1.6
112	Mango	34	59	253	0.5	0	15.3
113	Melon	40	23	97	0.8	0	5.2
114	Oranges	25	35	150	0.8	0	8.5
115	Orange juice	0	38	161	0.6	0	9.4
116	Peaches	13	37	156	0.6	0	9.1
117	Peaches, canned in syrup	0	87	373	0.4	0	22.9
118	Pears	28	41	175	0.3	0	10.6

[1] Old potatoes   [2] New potatoes

ter	Calcium mg	Iron mg	Sodium mg	Vitamin A (retinol equivalent) μg	Thia-min mg	Ribo-flavin mg	Niacin equivalent mg	Vitamin C mg	No.
5	23	0.3	13	0	0.04	0.04	0.3	8	77
2	13	2.4	12	3	0.11	0.04	1.6	0	78
5	23	0.9	9	167	0.07	0.08	0.4	15	79
2	3	1.0	9	0	0.10	0.40	4.6	3	80
3	31	0.3	10	0	0.03	0.05	0.4	10	81
3	36	0.5	4	0	0.07	0.06	0.9	10	82
3	35	1.6	2	50	0.30	0.09	1.6	12	83
)	33	1.8	380	10	0.10	0.04	1.4	0	84
1	9	0.4	2	33	0.08	0.03	0.9	100	85
)	8	0.4	8	0	0.20	0.02	1.5	8-19	86
●	4	0.4	7	0	0.20	0.02	1.2	5-9	87
3	37	2.1	550	0	0.19	0.07	6.1	17	88
1	14	0.84	41	0	0.2	0.02	1.5	6-14	89
)	1	0.8	53	0	0.1	0.04	3.1	12	90
5	10	0.62	9	0	0.2	0.02	1.3	5-12	91
5	136	4.0	120	1,000	0.07	0.15	1.8	25	92
2	4	0.5	270	4	0.04	0.06	1.8	0	93
●	22	0.7	19	4,000[3]	0.10	0.06	1.2	25	94
3	13	0.4	3	100	0.06	0.04	0.8	20	95
5	55	0.4	28	0	0.03	0.04	0.6	17	96
1	220	1.6	60	500	0.10	0.10	1.1	60	97
5	9	0.3	17	2	0.05	0.01	0.8	2	98
1	4	0.3	2	5	0.04	0.02	0.1	5	99
3	12	0.7	1	166	0.02	0.01	0.4	2	100
5	92	4.1	56	600	0	0.2	3.8	0	101
)	15	1.5	2	17	0.10	0.10	1.8	15	102
1	7	0.4	1	33	0.04	0.07	0.8	10	103
?	60	1.3	3	33	0.03	0.06	0.4	200	104
?	16	0.4	3	20	0.05	0.07	0.4	5	105
5	68	1.6	5	10	0.07	0.04	2.9	0	106
1	280	4.2	87	8	0.10	0.08	2.2	0	107
)	24	0.3	2	25	0.03	0.03	0.5	31	108
●	19	0.3	2	0	0.04	0.02	0.3	4	109
1	17	0.3	1	0	0.05	0.02	0.3	40	110
3	8	0.1	2	0	0.02	0.01	0.1	50	111
3	10	0.5	7	200	0.03	0.04	0.4	30	112
1	16	0.4	17	175	0.05	0.03	0.3	50	113
?	41	0.3	3	8	0.10	0.03	0.3	50	114
3	12	0.3	2	8	0.08	0.02	0.3	25-45	115
)	5	0.4	3	83	0.02	0.05	1.1	8	116
1	4	0.4	1	41	0.01	0.02	0.6	4	117
3	8	0.2	2	2	0.03	0.03	0.3	3	118

The vitamin A content of white and yellow varieties may vary between 0 and 12,000 μg

111

Composition per 100 g

No.	Food	Inedible waste %	Energy kcal	kJ	Protein g	Fat g	Carbohydrate (as monosaccharide) g
119	Pineapple, canned in juice	0	46	194	0.5	0	11.6
120	Plums	8	32	137	0.6	0	7.9
121	Prunes, dried	17	161	686	2.4	0	40.3
122	Raspberries	0	25	105	0.9	0	5.6
123	Rhubarb, cooked with sugar	0	45	191	0.5	0	11.4
124	Strawberries	3	26	109	0.6	0	6.2
125	Sultanas	0	250	1,066	1.8	0	64.7
	Nuts						
126	Almonds	63	565	2,336	16.9	53.5	4.3
127	Coconut, desiccated	0	604	2,492	5.6	62.0	6.4
128	Peanuts, roasted & salted	0	570	2,364	24.3	49.0	8.6
	Cereals						
129	Biscuits, chocolate	0	524	2,197	5.7	27.6	67.4
130	Biscuits, plain, digestive	0	471	1,978	6.3	20.9	68.6
131	Biscuits, semi-sweet	0	457	1,925	6.7	16.6	74.8
132	Bread, brown	0	217	924	8.4	2.0	44.2
133	Bread, white	0	230	980	8.2	1.7	48.6
134	Bread, wholemeal	0	215	911	9.0	2.5	41.6
	Breakfast cereals						
135	Cornflakes	0	368	1,567	8.6	1.6	85.1
136	Weetabix	0	340	1,444	11.4	3.4	70.3
137	Muesli	0	368	1,556	12.9	7.5	66.2
138	Cream crackers	0	440	1,857	9.5	16.3	68.3
139	Crispbread, rye	0	321	1,367	9.4	2.1	70.6
140	Flour, white	0	337	1,435	9.4	1.3	76.7
141	Flour, wholemeal	0	306	1,302	12.7	2.2	62.8
142	Oats, porridge	0	374	1,582	10.9	9.2	66.0
143	Rice, raw	0	359	1,529	7.0	1.0	85.8
144	Spaghetti, raw	0	342	1,456	12.0	1.8	74.1
	Cakes, etc						
145	Chocolate cake with butter icing	0	500	2,092	5.8	30.9	53.1
146	Currant buns	0	296	1,250	7.6	7.5	52.7
147	Fruit cake, rich	0	322	1,357	4.9	12.5	50.7
148	Jam tarts	0	368	1,552	3.3	13.0	63.4
149	Plain cake, Madeira	0	393	1,652	5.4	16.9	58.4
	Puddings						
150	Apple pie	0	369	1,554	4.3	15.5	56.7
151	Bread and butter pudding	0	157	661	6.1	7.7	16.9
152	Cheesecake, frozen, fruit topping	0	239	1,005	5.2	10.6	32.8
153	Custard	0	118	496	3.8	4.4	16.7

ater	Calcium	Iron	Sodium	Vitamin A (retinol equivalent)	Thia-min	Ribo-flavin	Niacin equivalent	Vitamin C	No.
	mg	mg	mg	µg	mg	mg	mg	mg	
′7	12	0.4	1	7	0.08	0.02	0.3	20-40	119
‹5	12	0.3	2	37	0.05	0.03	0.6	3	120
′3	38	2.9	12	160	0.10	0.20	1.9	0	121
‹3	41	1.2	3	13	0.02	0.03	0.5	25	122
‹5	84	0.3	2	8	0	0.03	0.4	7	123
‹9	22	0.7	2	5	0.02	0.03	0.5	60	124
8	52	1.8	53	5	0.10	0.08	0.6	0	125
5	250	4.2	6	0	0.24	0.92	4.7	0	126
2	22	3.6	28	0	0.06	0.04	1.8	0	127
5	61	2.0	440	0	0.23	0.10	21.3	0	128
2	110	1.7	160	0	0.03	0.13	2.7	0	129
5	92	3.2	600	0	0.14	0.11	2.4	0	130
5	120	2.1	410	0	0.13	0.08	2.9	0	131
0	99	2.2	540	0	0.27	0.10	2.3	0	132
8	105	1.6	525	0	0.21	0.06	2.3	0	133
8	54	2.7	560	0	0.34	0.09	1.8	0	134
0	3	6.7	1,160	0	1.8	1.6	21.9	0	135
8	33	7.6	360	0	1.0	1.5	14.3	0	136
8	200	4.6	180	0	0.33	0.27	5.7	0	137
3	110	1.7	610	0	0.13	0.08	3.4	0	138
4	50	3.7	220	0	0.28	0.14	2.9	0	139
0	140	2.0	2	0	0.31	0.04	3.5	0	140
0	38	3.9	2	0	0.47	0.09	8.3	0	141
2	52	3.8	9	0	0.90	0.09	3.3	0	142
4	4	0.5	4	0	0.41	0.02	5.8	0	143
8	25	2.1	3	0	0.22	0.03	3.1	0	144
4	130	1.6	440	298	0.07	0.09	2.0	0	145
7	110	1.9	230	0	0.37	0.16	3.1	0	146
6	84	3.2	220	0	0.07	0.09	1.3	0	147
4	72	1.7	130	0	0.06	0.02	1.2	0	148
2	42	1.1	380	0	0.06	0.11	1.6	0	149
9	51	1.2	210	0	0.05	0.02	0.4	0	150
5	130	0.6	150	78	0.07	0.23	1.8	0	151
0	68	0.5	160	0	0.04	0.16	1.7	0	152
9	140	0.1	76	38	0.05	0.20	1.0	0	153

113

Composition per 100 g

No.	Food	Inedible waste	Energy		Protein	Fat	Carbo-hydrate (as mono saccharic
		%	kcal	kJ	g	g	g
154	Ice cream, dairy	0	165	691	3.3	8.2	20.7
155	Rice pudding	0	131	552	4.1	4.2	20.4
156	Trifle	0	165	690	2.2	9.2	19.5
	Beverages						
157	Chocolate, drinking	0	366	1,554	5.5	6.0	77.4
158	Cocoa powder	0	312	1,301	18.5	21.7	11.5
159	Coffee, ground, infusion	0	3	12	0.3	0	0.4
160	Coffee, instant powder	0	100	424	14.6	0	11.0
161	Carbonated 'ades	0	38	166	0	0	10.0
162	Tea, dry	0	0	0	0	0	0
163	Squash, undiluted	0	98	418	0	0	26.1
	Alcoholic beverages						
164	Beer, keg bitter	0	37	156	0	0	2.3
165	Spirits	0	222	919	0	0	0
166	Wine, medium white	0	89	371	0	0	2.5
167	Cider, average	0	43	180	0	0	2.9
	Miscellaneous						
168	Curry powder	0	325	1,395	12.7	13.8	41.8
169	Marmite	0	179	759	41.4	0.7	1.8
170	Peanut butter	0	623	2,581	22.6	53.7	13.1
171	Soy sauce	0	56	240	5.2	0.5	8.3
172	Tomato soup	0	55	230	0.8	3.3	5.9
173	Tomato ketchup	0	98	420	2.1	0	24.0
174	Pickle, sweet	0	134	572	0.6	0.3	34.4
175	Salad cream	0	311	1,288	1.9	27.4	15.1

ter	Calcium	Iron	Sodium	Vitamin A (retinol equivalent)	Thia-min	Ribo-flavin	Niacin equivalent	Vitamin C	No.
	mg	mg	mg	μg	mg	mg	mg	mg	
7	120	0.3	70	0	0.04	0.15	0.9	0	154
3	30	0.1	55	33	0.04	0.14	1.1	0	155
1	68	0.3	63	50	0.06	0.10	0.6	0	156
2	33	2.4	2	2	0.06	0.04	2.1	0	157
3	130	10.5	7	7	0.16	0.06	7.3	0	158
3	3	0.1	1	0	0	0.01	0.6	0	159
3	140	4.6	81	0	0.04	0.21	27.9	0	160
1	4	0.1	8	0	0	0	0	0	161
9	0	0	0	0	0	0.9	6.0	0	162
2	11	0.1	35	0	0	0.01	0.1	5	163
3	8	0	6	0	0	0.03	0.17	0	164
4	0	0	0	0	0	0	0	0	165
5	10	0.4	1	0	0	0	0.1	0	166
2	5	0.2	7	0	0	0	0	0	167
	478	29.6	52	99	0.25	0.28	3.5	11	168
	95	3.7	4,500	0	3.10	11.0	67	0	169
	37	2.1	350	0	0.17	0.10	15	0	170
	65	4.8	5,720	0	0.04	0.17	1.8	0	171
4	17	0.4	460	35	0.03	0.02	0.6	0	172
5	25	1.2	1,120	0	0.06	0.05	0.3	0	173
	19	2.0	1,700	0	0.03	0.01	0.2	0	174
2.7	34	0.8	840	0	0	0	0	0	175

3 The use of food tables for calculations on the nutritional value of foods

A great deal of useful information can be worked out from the food composition tables in Appendix 2. Examples of various types of calculations are given below:

1. *NUTRIENT CONTENT*

(a) *Simple nutrient content*

To calculate the protein content of 2 *fish fingers*

Fish fingers (food no. 43) contain 12.6 g protein per 100 g

2 fish fingers weigh 56 g (Appendix 4)

$\therefore$ 56 g raw fish fingers contain $12.6 \times \dfrac{56}{100}$

$\qquad\qquad = 7.1$ g protein

(b) *Nutrient content allowing for wastage (inedible matter)*

To calculate the carbohydrate content of one *apple* weighing 120 g:

Apples (food no. 99) contain 11.9 g carbohydrate per 100 g edible portion, and 20 per cent waste.

A 120 g apple contains $\dfrac{100-20}{100} \times 120$ g edible matter

$\qquad\qquad = 96$ g edible matter

Therefore 120 g whole apple contains $\dfrac{96}{100} \times 11.9$

$\qquad\qquad = 11.4$ g carbohydrate

2. *PORTION SIZES*

(a) *100 kilocalorie portions*

e.g. *Cheddar cheese*

Cheddar cheese (food no. 10) has an energy value of 406 kcal per 100 g

$\therefore$ 100 kcal are contained in $\dfrac{100}{406} \times 100$

$\qquad\qquad = 25$ g (or just under 1 oz Cheddar cheese)

or *Cottage cheese*

Cottage cheese (food no. 11) has an energy value of 96 kcal per 100 g

$\therefore$100 kcal are contained in $\dfrac{100}{96} \times 100$

$$= 104 \text{ g (or just under 4 oz) cottage cheese}$$

(b) *400 kilojoule portions* (The size of a 400 kJ portion will be slightly smaller than a 100 kcal portion, while a 500 kJ portion will be larger) eg, *Egg*

Eggs (food no. 50) have an energy value of 612 kJ per 100 g edible portion

$\therefore$400 kJ are contained in $\dfrac{400}{612} \times 100$

$$= 65 \text{ g egg}$$

Since eggs contain 12 per cent inedible material (shell), this is equivalent to:

$65 \times \dfrac{100}{100-12}$ $= 74$ g of egg in its shell.

(c) *Portion sizes in relation to recommended daily amounts of nutrients*
To calculate the amount of *beef supplying one sixth of the recommended daily amount (RDA) of iron* for girls aged 15-17.

One sixth of the RDA = 2 mg (p 56)

Beef (food no. 17) contains 1.9 mg iron per 100 g edible portion

$\therefore$2 mg are contained in $\dfrac{2.0}{1.9} \times 100$

$$= 105.3 \text{ g edible beef}$$

To convert from grams to ounces

28.35 g = 1 oz

$\therefore 105.3$ g $= \dfrac{105.3}{28.35} = 3.71$ oz beef

3. COST OF NUTRIENTS

(a) *Nutrients per penny*

To calculate the nutrients obtained per penny from a large (800 g) loaf of *white bread* costing 48p

1p buys $\dfrac{1}{48} \times 800$

$$= 16.7 \text{ g}$$

Item no. 133 shows the nutrients in 100 g white bread. Therefore multiply the values for each nutrient by $\dfrac{16.7}{100}$

$$= 1.4 \text{ g protein}$$
$$= 0.3 \text{ g fat}$$
$$= 8.1 \text{ g carbohydrate}$$
$$= 17.5 \text{ mg calcium}$$
$$= 0.3 \text{ mg iron, etc}$$

(b)   To calculate the cost of 10 g protein from *baked beans*
Baked beans (food no. 65) contain 4.8 g protein per 100 g

$\therefore$10 g protein are contained in $\dfrac{10}{4.8} \times 100$

$$= 208.3 \text{ g baked beans}$$

At a cost of 25p per 450 g can

208.3 g of baked beans cost $\dfrac{208.3}{450} \times 25$

$$= 11.6 \text{ pence}$$

4. PERCENTAGE OF ENERGY FROM FAT

(a)   *In a food* such as *brown bread*
Brown bread (food no. 132) contains 2.0 g fat and 217 kcals (924 kJ) per 100 g

$\therefore$One large slice (30 g) contains $\dfrac{30}{100} \times 217$ kcals

$$= 65.1 \text{ kcals (or 277.2 kJ)}$$

and $\dfrac{30}{100} \times 2.0$ g fat

$$= 0.60 \text{ g fat}$$

Each gram of fat provides 9 kcals or 37 kJ

$\therefore$The percentage of energy from fat $= \dfrac{0.60 \times 9}{65.1} \times 100 = 8.3\%$

$$\left(\text{or } \dfrac{0.6 \times 37}{277.2} \times 100 = 8.0\% \right)$$

or *Butter*
Butter (food no. 52) contains 82.0 g fat and 740 kcals (3,041 kJ) per 100 g
Allowing 7 g butter for a slice of bread;

7 g butter contains $\dfrac{7 \times 740}{100}$ kcals

$$= 51.8 \text{ kcals (or 212.9 kJ)}$$

and $\dfrac{7 \times 8.20}{100}$ g fat

$$= 5.74 \text{ g fat}$$

$\therefore$The percentage of energy from fat $= \dfrac{5.74 \times 9}{51.8} \times 100 = 99.7\%$

$$\left(\text{or } \dfrac{5.74 \times 37}{212.9} = 99.8\% \right)$$

(b)   *In a combination of foods*
One slice of bread (30 g) and butter (7 g) contains 0.6 + 5.74 g fat (see examples above)

$$= 6.34 \text{ g fat}$$

and 65.1 + 51.8 kcals   = 116.9 kcal

or   277.2 + 212.9 kJ   = 490.1 kJ

Since each gram of fat provides 9 kcals or 37 kJ the percentage of energy from fat in a slice of bread and butter is

$$\frac{6.34 \times 9 \times 100}{116.9} = 48.8\%$$

$$(\text{or } \frac{6.34 \times 37 \times 100}{490.1} = 47.9\%)$$

Adding jam (or a drink) would further reduce the proportion of energy derived from fat.

N.B. The values derived from kilocalories and kilojoules differ slightly since the conversion factors given on page 104 are not exactly equivalent.

4 Approximate servings of commonly used foods

Milk	for { 1 cup of tea	28 g
	{ 1 glass	200 g
Cheese	'matchbox-sized' piece	50 g
Pork chop	medium size, raw	180 g
Minced beef	average portion, raw	120 g
Bacon	large rasher, raw	40 g
Sausage	large sausage, raw	55 g
Meat pie	individual pie	130 g
Fish finger	1 fish finger	28 g
Egg	size 3	60-64 g
Butter, margarine or low fat spread	for 1 slice bread	7-10 g
Lettuce	2 large leaves	15 g
Potatoes, boiled	2 medium	120 g
mashed	1 scoop	60 g
Orange	medium sized (with peel)	120 g
Apple	medium sized	120 g
Bread	{ medium slice from small loaf	25 g
	{ medium slice from large loaf	30 g
Flour	1 tablespoon, rounded	30 g
Porridge oats	1 teacup	80 g
Breakfast cereal	1 helping	20-30 g
Crispbread	1 crispbread	14 g
Biscuits, digestive	1 biscuit	14 g
Rice	2 heaped tablespoons, boiled	60 g
Coffee, instant	per cup	2-3 g
Tea	per cup	5 g
Sugar	1 teaspoon	5 g
Beer	½ pint	285 g (285 ml)
Wine	1 wineglass	120 g (120 ml)

5 Food additives

In addition to the expected ingredients of made-up foods there are other substances which may be added in small amounts to perform a special function in the food. These are called *food additives*. They fall into two broad categories: those which are added to prevent food spoilage and those which are added to enhance the texture, flavour or appearance of food.

Preservatives and antioxidants

It is very important that every effort is made to prevent sound food being wasted. Some forms of food spoilage, such as attacks on stored food by vermin, are easily recognized. Other forms of spoilage develop within the food itself and give rise to off-flavours long before the visual appearance of the food itself is noticeably affected; these may arise either by the action of micro-organisms (i.e., moulds and bacteria) or by chemical action. While some micro-organisms merely make the food unpalatable, others such as *Clostridium botulinum* produce highly poisonous toxins and present a considerable hazard to health. Preservatives such as sulphur dioxide and sodium nitrite are added to some foods to inhibit the growth of micro-organisms. The most common form of chemical spoilage is rancidity. Rancidity resulting from the oxidation of fat can be retarded by the addition of antioxidants. Some antioxidants are natural compounds but in order to protect fat in foods which are baked, e.g. biscuits, heat-stable synthetic antioxidants are required.

Other additives

The texture of food often depends on the ability of added emulsifiers to form a uniform dispersion of fat and water e.g., in margarine and salad cream. Similarly, stabilizers are added to prevent uniform dispersions separating out e.g., in the setting of instant desserts.

The colour and flavour of foods are closely linked: consumers expect a food to have a colour which matches the flavour. Therefore, if the natural colour is lost or changed during processing, colouring matter may be added to restore the food to the expected colour.

The law strictly controls the additives which may be used in food (see also Appendix 6), and the list of ingredients must show the name or where appropriate the category name or serial number of any additives used in the food (e.g. E300, ascorbic acid, or 500, sodium bicarbonate).

6   Legislation governing the composition and labelling of food

The major piece of legislation in this field is the *Food Act 1984*. Legislation is made jointly by the Minister of Agriculture and the Secretary of State for Social Services. This applies only in England and Wales, but there is similar legislation in Scotland and Northern Ireland.

The most important provisions of the Act are: (a) to make it an offence to sell to the prejudice of the purchaser food which is not of the nature, substance or quality demanded, (b) to prohibit the use of a label or advertisement which falsely describes a food or misleads as to its nature, substance or quality, (c) to prohibit the addition to or abstraction of any substance from food so as to render the food injurious to health, and (d) make it an offence to sell unsound food. These general provisions are backed up by many regulations which lay down detailed requirements as to the labelling of all foods, the composition of the major foods (as below) in our diet, and the type and level of additives and contaminants permitted in food.

Ministers are advised on the need for and type of regulations by the Food Advisory Committee which consults all interested parties, including consumers, enforcement officers and the food industries before coming to any decisions. Before making regulations, Ministers are again required to consult all those interested.

The Food Labelling Regulations 1984 require most prepacked foods to bear a common or usual name or an appropriate designation of the food, a list of ingredients in descending order by weight, the name and address of the packer or labeller (or somebody resident in the United Kingdom who is responsible for the food), and an indication of the minimum durability of the food. These regulations also set strict conditions which must be followed before there can be a claim on the label or in advertising that, for example, the food will provide energy or protein, is an aid to slimming, or will be useful to diabetics. Vitamin and mineral claims may only be made for the following nutrients: vitamin A, thiamin, riboflavin, niacin, folic acid, vitamin B_{12}, vitamin C, vitamin D, calcium, iodine and iron.

The compositional regulations lay down standards for certain foods; for example, minimum meat contents are linked to certain permitted names in the meat products regulations. A pork sausage, for instance, under the *Meat Product and Spreadable Fish Product Regulations 1984* must contain 65 per cent meat but a beef sausage only 50 per cent.

Detailed requirements are laid down for the composition of bread by the

Bread and Flour Regulations 1984. The use of colouring matter is restricted, the permitted bleaching and improving agents listed, minimum nutrient levels for flour are prescribed, and the amount of chalk which must be added to all flour except self-raising, wholemeal and wheat malt flour laid down (see also page 80).

The *Margarine Regulations 1967* require, amongst other things, that all margarine for retail sale must be fortified with vitamins A and D and that this must be declared on the label (see also page 72).

The additive regulations lay down lists of permitted additives and standards of purity. The safety of additives and the need for their use are given full and detailed consideration before they are permitted to be used in food. Existing regulations control, for example, preservatives, colouring matters, antioxidants, and emulsifiers and stabilizers. Food contaminants such as heavy metals are also strictly controlled by legislation.

The full Regulations, which are obtainable from Her Majesty's Stationery Office, should be consulted for further information, but a brief account of the labelling regulations, including a complete list of additive serial numbers, is also available from the Ministry of Agriculture, Fisheries and Food *(Look at the Label)*. Another free leaflet giving additive names and numbers only is also available.

7 Books for further reading

W Matthews and D Wells. *Second Book of Food and Nutrition*. 3rd ed. Home Economics and Flour Advisory Bureau, London: 1976. £6.50.

(ISBN 0 90 176223 7)

M Pyke. *Success in Nutrition*. London: John Murray, 1982. £3.25.

(ISBN 0 71 953186 1)

Sir S Davidson, R Passmore, J F Brock and A S Truswell. *Human Nutrition and Dietetics*. 7th ed. Edinburgh: Churchill Livingstone, 1979. £18.00.

(ISBN 0 44 307310 1)

Department of Health and Social Security. *Eating for Health*. London: HMSO, 1978. £2.50.

(ISBN 0 11 320665 8)

The Health Education Council. *Proposals for Nutritional Guidelines for Health Education in Britain*. (NACNE). London: 1983. Free publication from the Health Education Council.

Department of Health and Social Security. *Present Day Practice in Infant Feeding*. Report on Health and Social Subjects No. 20. London: HMSO, 1980. £4.15.

(ISBN 0 11 320749 2)

Department of Health and Social Security. *Diet and Cardiovascular Disease*. Report on Health and Social Subjects No. 28. London: HMSO, 1984. £3.35.

(ISBN 0 11 3208596)

Department of Health and Social Security. *Recommended Daily Amounts of Food Energy and Nutrients for Groups of People in the UK*. Report on Health and Social Subjects No. 15. London: HMSO, 1979. £2.70.

(ISBN 0 11 320342 X)

US National Research Council Food and Nutrition Board. *Recommended Dietary Allowances*. 9th revised ed. Washington: National Academy of Sciences 1980.

(ISBN 0 309 02941 1)

B Nilson. *Cooking for Special Diets*. 3rd ed. Harmondsworth: Penguin. 1981. £3.95.

(ISBN 0 14 046095 0)

L R Brown. *By Bread Alone*. Overseas Development Council. Pergamon Press, 1975. £6.50.

(ISBN 0 08 019946)

J C Drummond and A Wilbraham. *The Englishman's Food:* A History of Five Centuries of English Diet. 2nd ed. London: Jonathan Cape, 1958.

(ISBN 0 22 460168 7)

Ministry of Agriculture, Fisheries and Food. *Household Food Consumption and Expenditure.* Annual Reports of the National Food Survey Committee. London: HMSO.

A E Bender. *Dictionary of Nutrition and Food Technology.* 5th ed. London: Newnes-Butterworth, 1982. £17.50. (ISBN 0 40 800143 7)

A E Bender. *Food Processing and Nutrition.* London: Academic Press, 1978. £33.50. (ISBN 0 12 086450 9)

A A Paul and D A T Southgate. McCance and Widdowson's *The Composition of Foods.* 4th ed. London: HMSO, 1978. £18.00.

(ISBN 0 11 450036 3)

S P Tan, R W Wenlock and D H Buss. *Immigrant Foods.* London: HMSO, 1985. £4.50. (ISBN 0 11 242717 0)

United States Department of Agriculture. *Composition of Foods Raw, Processed and Prepared.* Agriculture Handbook No. 8, parts 1-13. Washington, 1976-1985.

Index

128

Printed in the UK for HMSO

Dd 738266 C300 8/85